Fifty and Beyond

New Beginnings in Health and Well-Being

What people are saying

"This book is pure joy! Susanna avoids lecturing, but instead opens up possibilities in the areas of health, lifestyle changes and spirituality. She encourages the reader to think, to experiment and to assume responsibility for creating a joyful life and she suggests reasonable ways to accomplish this."
– SUSAN BACHRACH, owner, Moby Dickens Bookshop,

"… Susanna Starr has a way of helping us to see that growing older is a privilege and a gift to be shared. After reading *Fifty and Beyond*, I feel like aging is something to look forward to!"
– PAULINA LITTLE, *Third Ager's Magazine*,

"*Fifty and Beyond* is a meditation on aging. Neither a lament nor a complaint, Susanna Starr writes with compassion, concern, joy, and enthusiasm about how we choose to live the last years of our life. I highly recommend this book to anyone who is willing to open their minds and their hearts to new life-long possibilities.
– NANCY KING, PH.D., author of *Giving Form to Feeling* and many other books and articles

"Written with the kind of passion for life one discovers through rigorous introspection Susanna Starr's *Fifty and Beyond: New Beginnings in Health and Well-Being* provides a long list of wise and doable ways in which to muster mind, body and soul in the battle against old age. It's must reading for anyone thinking about becoming (gasp!) 'elderly.'"
– JOHN K WHITNEY, Editor, *Taos Magazine*

"What a wonderful gift! Susanna helps us all shift the prospect of aging from a fear of the unknown to the anticipation of pleasure. Thank you!"
–AIMEE LYNDON-ADAMS, business consultant, keynote speaker

"You're never too old to be young. Susanna Starr shows us how to enjoy the best part of our lives physically, emotionally and spiritually. – A joyous perspective of life's treasures and how to maximize your journey."
– LARRY SCHREIBER, M.D., family physician

Fifty and Beyond
New Beginnings in Health and Well-Being

Susanna Starr

Paloma Blanca Press • Taos, New Mexico USA

Fifty and Beyond
New Beginnings in Health and Well-Being
by Susanna Starr

Published by:
Paloma Blanca Press
info@PalomaBlancaPress.com
877-520-4890
PO Box 1751, Taos, NM 87571 USA

Starr, Susanna.
    Fifty and beyond: new beginnings in health and well-being / by Susanna Starr. -- 1st ed.
    p. cm.
    Includes bibliographical reference and index.
    LCCN 2002105566
    ISBN 0-9720084-4-6

    1. Middle aged persons--United States--Life skills guides. 2. Aged--United States--Life skills guides.
    1. Title.

HQ1059.5.U5S83 2002   646.7'0084'4
                                     QBI33-633

Cover & book design by Cowgirls Design, Taos, New Mexico
Cover art by Marjory Reid
Photographs by Saskia Van Der Lingen
Printed in the United States of America
First edition
08 07 06 05 04 03   8 7 6 5 4 3 2 1
Printed on acid free paper

"The best is yet to come."

– GABOO (TED THOMAS),
Australian aboriginal elder

Contents

Acknowledgements

I think part of my reason for writing this book is to thank all the people in print that I do in my heart for all they've given to me, for providing the love and the richness that has spun the warp on which is woven the weft of my life.

To the loving memory of my oldest son, Matthew, who chose to spend the brief ten and a half years of his life with us as his family and with me as his mother. To my beautiful children, Mirabai, Amy and Roy, who have given me the deepest joy a mother could know and who are my closest friends. In spite of my falling short of being the "perfect mother" each young woman expects to be with her children, they have developed on their own to be the superb human beings I not only love but honor and respect.

To my grandsons, Nicholas and Ian, who have put up with years of lectures and sermons on the mount, and who still ask for bedtime stories even when they know it's going to deal with some kind of "moral." To my granddaughter, Daniela, who is now the beautiful young mother of Jacob and Breanna. And to the loving memory of Jenny, my other granddaughter, who is recently gone from our lives, but like Matty, never from our hearts and memories.

To the men in my life. First, my father, who was "Daddy" to me until the day he died. He taught me to whistle, to tie my shoelaces, to tell time, to sing and recite epic poetry before I was five years old. He sang with me, taught me to play softball, took me fishing and berry picking. From him I learned my love of the land and how to garden. His ever present smile and sense of humor, gentleness and caring have always been "what I came home to," whether as part of the household or many years later with miles in-between. He told me outrageous stories when I was a child. He never complained when he was dying.

He gave to my children all that he gave to me, including changing their diapers and giving them bottles. His way was not the way of ambition, of acquisition (I still have the tool box of many years that he left on his kitchen table when he checked himself into the hospital just before he died – I knew they were meant for me to have and to take care of as he had always done). His needs were simple – reading or playing in the garden, eating basically, living quietly, avoiding stress because that was his nature, loving his family. Although he's no longer living, the memories that have nurtured me continue.

To Ian, my husband and the father of my four children. Although we had not lived together for almost twenty years, our abiding connection remained until the day he died. We shared our family together, our early years of marriage, raising our children, somehow surviving the loss of our oldest, being young together and learning what it meant to take on the responsibilities and joys of young adulthood. Although the form changed, the love remained.

To John, for his quiet and calmness, who has provided me with a safe haven, the space to find my own centeredness, the place within myself that has made it possible to write this book. He continues to "be there" for me, providing support, companionship and harmony.

To all the men in my life who have loved me, and in loving me, have given me support, my all the time friends. I love your strengths and thank you for seeing mine.

To my mother and all the women who have been, and continue to be, in my life. So many, so beautiful! I'm forever grateful to have been born into a woman's body, to be part of this sacred sisterhood that provides the love and support for each other as well as for their children, for their men, in a way only a woman can know and appreciate. The strength that has so often been honed as the result of pain, suffering and exploitation, the caring for and about those for whom they have assumed the mantle of responsibility which lays wrapped around their sometimes fragile shoulders, their willingness to grow and share, to create, should be an inspiration not only to other women, but men as well.

To all the people I've worked with, many of whom I

continue to work with, most over many years. For making that "work" time, another aspect of "life" time. In sharing so many hours together, I have found enrichment through caring and humor. Their feeling of involvement and connection has made that part of my life an easier and nicer one.

And to the Universe for what it's given me. I've slept on the beach and in cars. I've lived without indoor plumbing and running water. I've chopped wood and carried water. I've built lots of fires. I've lived on food stamps and know what it's like not to have enough money to give to your child for something as simple as an ice-cream cone. I've spent many years working seven days a week and not being with my children during some of the most precious times of their lives, as children. I've known the numbness of loss, the sadness of the void in my life. But I have always been blessed with the most important things that life has to offer, surrounded by beauty and filled and nurtured by love. I am eternally grateful for the eyes with which to see and the heart with which to receive.

Special thanks to those who helped me put this book together – my daughter, Mirabai, for taking on the job of editing when she was so immersed in her own writing, with deadlines to meet. My partner, John Lamkin for the months and months of research on publishing and marketing, whose ideas on layout and presentation are evident throughout this book, whose quiet confidence that it would come to fruition, have provided the launching pad. To Cowgirls Design for creating the book cover and book design. To Marjory Reid, a new friend in my life, whose inspiring painting appears on the book cover. To Jane Jeffries for putting the glossary together and for all the years spent in helping me keep my head screwed on straight. To Catherine Naylor for her help on the manuscript and to all my staff at La Unica Cosa and the Starr Gallery for making the time possible for me to do it!

Also many thanks to Graham Nash, Paulina Little, Susan Bachrach, Jack Whitney, Nancy King, Larry Schreiber,

Aimee Lyndon-Adams and Linda Sparrowe. Thank you to those special people whose words appear on these pages: Dale Amburn, Helen Ambramowitz, Pat and Bill Stallcup, Ted Egri, Ann St. John Hawley and Tom Morrow.

Preface

"Grow old along with me, the best is yet to be." This line from a Robert Browning poem has always been one of my favorites.

From the time I was a teenager, I was fascinated by the idea of old age. The prospect of aging, with life having already unfolded, held a romantic lure for me. This poetic phrase seemed to reflect the promise of something very special. Was it a sense of some kind of reward, based on a different understanding, a measure of wisdom that would reveal itself as I got older, that held a special appeal to me when I was barely at the age of discovery of myself?

Now that I am in my sixties, I am even more aware of the gift of older people in my life. Since I first had the idea of writing this book, that value has become especially significant. Role models have always been important in every society, but in the prevailing culture of our time, the elderly are seldom respected or revered, but generally thought of as a segment of the population that does not "contribute" in the way of the "elders" of former times.

As time went by and the notion of writing this book on health and well-being became more of an imperative, it expanded on its own to include the accounts of a number of people who I felt were inspirational. Some of these people I had known for a long time, while others I didn't really know much at all, except for brief encounters in limited circumstances. Most of these people were in their mid to late eighties. All were people I admired for their spirit, for their attitude about how they chose to live their lives. The thing they had in common was that they worked at maintaining their strength, vitality and creativity. Their positive attitude made them appear younger than their years, or rather, evoked a feeling that did not necessarily relate to chronological age.

Not only were these older people a source of inspiration but I recognized in many of my own friends the same attitudes and life styles that placed them, too, at an unidentifiable age.

The hallmark of all these people is their energy and vitality. In every case, they see themselves being in charge of their own lives and are consciously working on maintaining a state of well-being, active and involved in life.

After experiencing one of my own personal transformations when I was just past sixty, I became excited about what can happen when we take control of our own bodies and minds. Taking what could have been a negative situation and watching it transform into something positive was liberating. What had begun as a traumatic time for me became simply a way to go beyond the circumstances, and to work with my inner self in order for that self to become more expansive.

Without any thought, but as the most natural form of expression, I began immediately to journal, something I had not done since my high school days. While my thoughts and emotions were fresh, I documented my own experience and found that my old writing tool was still of great value, in spite of the years of non-use. Those years had been focused on working, raising a family, making significant life style changes, opening up ways of experiencing personal growth, and generally "being" rather than "recording."

As well as working on my internal self, now was a time when I could concentrate once again on my physical body which I had long taken for granted. That was an obvious place to influence change, since I realized that I needed to pay more attention to the way my body was serving me, as well as watch the internal process take place. Several months after I began my journal, I wrote one day "I'm getting my body back again – can my spirit be far behind?"

I began to see that all the work I was doing externally, through exercise, proper diet, and the use of supplements, was manifesting in a stronger, healthier, lighter body. As I opened up to make space to receive on the physical level, I felt my spirit once again become more fully realized as well. The stronger and more free I became through nurturing that inner self, the more open and receptive I was to explore different aspects of that self. Studying sculpture again after a lapse of many years got my creative juices flowing in a new way. Reading, which had always been such an important part of my life but had been relegated to the "back burner" because of what I had perceived as a lack of time, became a food, and I devoured books as if to make up for all the years without. Much came pouring in through different sources, and I felt myself "waking up" again, something that was a very familiar feeling.

We have a tendency when we hear the phrase "fitness" to think of physical fitness. This, however, is just one part of well-being. Having a body that's strong and flexible, providing stamina and endurance takes work. Keeping our immune system functioning at a high level, which might prevent us from entertaining every itinerant form of bacteria seeking residency in our bodies, requires constant diligence. Our minds, too, need exercise to expand our understanding of the options that are open to us. We can be more discriminating in our choices of how we receive information so that we can be better and more wisely informed. We can break out of former, more limited patterns, using a firm foundation of solid judgment, using our own information rather than that which is imposed upon us. This, too, is an integral part of overall fitness.

With a sound body and mind, the spiritual connection we each seek, whether consciously or not, will naturally present itself for what we are as human beings is an integrated whole. That means the parts working harmoniously together. In so doing, we not only do the best we can by maintaining a high standard of fitness on all levels but also allow ourselves the opportunity and space to receive what the Universe has to offer. I've found that all I do to keep myself physically fit, emotionally centered, and spiritually connected is not work but is itself the reward. The feeling of accomplishing what I consider to be my real work provides me with that sense of fulfillment of self I believe we each search for.

Introduction

hether or not you believe you might live to be one hundred and that you still have almost half of your life ahead of you, or feel you might fall somewhat short of that life span, now can be a great time to begin a serious program of fitness. This is a critical phase of life and what we do to take care of ourselves now may mean the difference in the way we spend our later years. It can result in those years finding us able to utilize our life force and energy level to give us the quality of life we'd like to have, or spending those years in decline, mentally, physically and spiritually.

If this book has captured your attention because you thought it would give you an exercise program, tell you what and how to eat, provide fabulous recipes for healthy foods or reveal an exciting and innovative program for a long life, please put it down now and don't waste your time. It will not provide answers, nor will it specifically address questions such as "how can I ...?". It's not for those who are looking for another form of instant gratification; how to get and stay in wonderful shape, look like the models on magazine covers, be forever young. As a matter of fact, the thoughts expressed here are in direct opposition to these concepts. Rather, it's about embracing and nurturing the best of who you already are without trying to replace yourself with a new model. Often those ideas are not only unattainable and unrealistic, but focus more on appearance than substance.

Approaching fifty often seems to represent a major milestone in our lives. Perhaps it's because we feel we've completed the first half and are uncertain about what to do about the next part. For many, it's a time of major re-evaluation and for some, a sense of dislocation. For most people, growing older used to be understood as part of a natural process. In many societies it was a time when work and struggle gave way to a more tranquil time to enjoy some of the fruits of their labor. In many societies, the elders were actually revered!

If you've read this far, may I encourage you to celebrate where you are now, approaching mid-life, or well into it. What a wonderful, exciting and joyous time it is and how blessed we are to realize how much more there can to be, and how much better equipped we are to recognize and enjoy it. Do you look into the mirror and smile at who you see reflected there? Do you love those same features you were so critical of when you were young and caught up in the way you "should" look or would like to look? Can you see that the lines in your face represent so many of your life's experiences, laughter and joy, sadness and grief, humor and compassion, worry and fear, gentleness and, perhaps, a little hint of wisdom? Or do you see hair that is graying that you think you should color, wrinkles that need makeup as a camouflage, sagging muscles and loosening skin that tell you in no uncertain terms, you're no longer thirty-five. How wonderful! I've already been thirty-five. I've also been twenty-five. Not only do I not have to be there again, I don't have to look the same way as I did then.

Surely, by now, we understand that everything changes and in so doing evolves into different forms. How exciting! How liberating not to be tied into a fixed structure, but one that is in constant flux. Like many people I know, I feel that I've lived at least several different lives already in this particular lifetime and as much as I've changed on a physical level, so have I also undergone other forms of transformation and, I hope, significant growth on other levels as well.

Section One
The Shift

The Universe is not static

But always in a state of flux

So, too, we are always shifting

And changing, realigning

Chapter One
The Program Begins

*I*f you've not yet consciously begun a program that will enable you to wake up to a state of awareness that engages your mind, body and spirit, now's the time to begin. For so long, we've been occupied with educating ourselves, finding a job, establishing a career, raising a family, building a home, cultivating a life with all its responsibilities, dealing with relationships, exploring opportunities, growing and maturing, learning from others and from our own experiences, that we've often left the introspective part of ourselves to simmer quietly on the back burner. Isn't it exciting to think of all that is opening up to us at this stage of our lives? It should and could be a time of joy and celebration, of contem-

"Every painting I start is an adventure. The only thing I have limiting me when I start a painting is the canvas ... the composition, the color relationships, the forms and everything relate to the first thing I do on canvas ... I paint because I see things or I think of things that I want to see on canvas, and they touch me, they make me feel good, so I try to put them down on canvas for a message for other people. My diary hangs on the wall ... I hang myself naked on the wall."

– DALE AMBURN

"I never felt resentful because I always took a morning off to do something, to go and do art, sing, study piano, dance – my spirit was always involved."

"You have to have your own world."

– ANN ST. JOHN HAWLEY

"I feel that we have to create our own lives – I think your attitude is the most important thing you have."

"It's very important to have a purpose – to stay healthy, keep the house, create things, read. Without purpose, you can fade away, die."

– HELEN ABRAMOWITZ

plation and reflection, of finding comfort in the discovery of who we are and our relation to our Universe. Ideally, this is a time of guiding others along their paths when we can be of service in a positive, healthy, non-imposing way, a way that is based on compassion and understanding. It's an invitation to open our hearts and share, whether it's time, experience or attention, and that includes to ourselves as well.

Many people, as they approach fifty (which is, of course, an arbitrary number of years), seem to be well aware of things like financial security, investments, monetary rewards such as pensions, investments and holdings of various kinds that will give them some kind of return and ensure some measure of ease as they look down the road toward aging. That's perfectly valid on one level, but surely there's much more we can do for ourselves. One obvious place we might think of focusing on is health and longevity. Living until one hundred may sound pretty good, and even somewhat reasonable, but what's quantity if it's lacking in quality? There are a number of things we can be doing right now, if we haven't already begun, to make that investment in our own health – body, mind and spirit. To begin a conscious program now can open new horizons, for as we find ourselves with increased energy and vitality our image of ourselves grows and our confidence in what this next half of our lives might offer expands.

This requires a real shift in consciousness for many people. In a society focused on the external and the emphasis placed on youth, many people, if they're able, like to do whatever they can to look young, act young, be "desirable and attractive." But looking good is not the same as being healthy. For the man who wants to slim down his waistline, which seems to have slowly expanded over the years, and decides to start working out at a health club, this is a good beginning. For the woman who wants to get back to the same size she was thirty years ago and starts an exercise routine, that's always a good start as well.

And if that's the way it begins for you, it's a positive move because at least you've placed yourself on a good path. But if you've done no more than talk about "getting into shape one of these days," I hope this book will inspire you to get going and do something meaningful for yourself. You might be pleasantly surprised to see the rewards that living consciously can do for you. These years can be some of the most rewarding in our lives, and one of the ways we can insure that, is to be aware right now of how to best take care of ourselves, so that later on, ideally, others won't have to do that for us.

How often have we heard of or dealt with the term, "midlife crisis?" It's as significant a threshold as puberty, when there's also a major shift in the maturation process. Most societies acknowledge these shifts with rituals. But how about that mid-age thing, what's the ritual there? Perhaps for the male of contemporary society, it's buying a new sports car (for the affluent), or finding a new young girlfriend (the non affluent can and do use this one as well). For the female, a sporty new car might not be satisfying, and a young boyfriend rarely holds much appeal. Maybe for her it's the constant quest for new lotions and potions guaranteed to "make you look young" (My favorite is the ad for wrinkle cream, using an eighteen year old as a model). Or dressing in the latest "fashion" which may not be terribly becoming on a seventy year old body.

The more serious and constructive side of this coin is that it can be a time of re-evaluation, in the most meaningful way, a way that expands and enhances this time of our lives. We often find ourselves raising questions such as "Where am I going from here? Do I have what it takes to make changes, to seek alternatives, to see things differently?" It involves a new commitment that requires incentive as well as faith. But as we increase our own strength, both inner and outer, we'll find that we have more of it for family and friends as well. And as we make new choices and find new directions, our increased sense of well-being is not only self rewarding but an inspiration to others.

As we open to the possibilities of new things in our lives, including friendships and creative expressions, we open ourselves through our hearts, rather than our minds, with more of an attitude of receiving that which is presented, rather than focusing on direction and control through excessive planning and incessant thinking. With letting go of the latter, we'll find ourselves much looser, more joyful, radiating that joy outward, as we discover the beauty of our own inner selves.

Chapter Two
A Shift in Time

*N*ow can be a time of indulgence and reward, but in a way different from that which you may have been programmed all your life to expect. An indulgence might now take the form of a "self-help" care program. If you embark on a program of this nature, it becomes not work but provides satisfaction in the most meaningful way. The transformation of mind, body and spirit, which will take place, is the most rewarding of all. We've been encouraged to focus on external things, on achievement, on success. But many of us have found that the old symbols of reward are empty and simply won't do any more. Now we can focus on feelings of achievement and success, but on a different level.

"I like to do things for people and I appreciate it when they do things for me. I can give a lot of my energy to other people – there's joy in giving, in doing, pleasure in giving to others."

– HELEN ABRAMOWITZ

Giving is always a joy when it's done with an open heart, no strings attached, which is to say, with no expectations. This is the only way it's an authentic action. This also applies to giving to ourselves, without guilt but with joy and reverence, as well as giving to others. We've learned a lot, and it's important to be able to share some of that knowledge we've obtained through our experiences. It can be rewarding to see how an insight can be transmitted to someone else who can apply it to a problem in their own lives. It sometimes can make a positive difference in how they treat what they considered to be an issue unique to themselves, by providing a broader perspective. Just be careful it's not preaching or imposing upon someone else, but simply presented. If they want to pick it up and use it, that's great, but no attachment on our part as to the outcome need be involved.

Which brings us to the most important part of all, which is spiritual consciousness. We might like to think this is a natural process of "living in the world," but that's not always the case. It often takes a deliberate shift to find our connection to that part of ourselves, and in so doing, to everything else. But when we do find ourselves with insights, an occasional revelation or two, and, the rarest of them all, an epiphany of sorts, how wonderful it is when we can radiate that outward, not necessarily through doing but by being.

"True values are much more simple - people, friends, love of family, the tranquility of living in a beautiful area with clean air and trees."

– HELEN ABRAMOWITZ

It's taken me until now to find myself taking the time simply to "be," letting go (at least sometimes) of the focus on what I think I need to "do." There are always things to do, to be taken care of and sometimes even what we consider leisure time can be filled with more emphasis on "doing" rather than on being able to open up the time and space to

"I'm not sure I'm going to get there, I have a way to go - the getting there is the exciting part!"

– ANN ST. JOHN HAWLEY

receive what is being offered to us. One of my greatest joys in these moments of my life is simply watching, hearing, smelling and just being present to what's going on around me. Sitting by our pond I can't help but be aware of the difference in the sounds of the various wind chimes, of the birdcalls, of the sound of the breeze in the trees. It's become a joyous time of serenity for me to just sit and watch the birds approach the water trickling down the rocks into the pond, to notice the way the sunlight hits different parts of the garden, to see what's newly budded and blooming. The perfume of the lilies is much more enthralling than anything to be sampled at a perfume counter!

"You have to have your own world."

This can be a time of focusing inward, of making a place for emptiness, of putting aside the mind's clutter and chatter, and of allowing myself the luxury of being in the moment rather than thinking and planning moments,

"The most important thing is your children – I had my dedication to my family and this secret place that was always roaming free."

– ANN ST. JOHN HAWLEY

days or weeks in the future. The more I find myself doing this, the easier it becomes. I still plan meetings, oversee projects, make commitments, but the commitment I've made to myself has begun to become the most significant task of all.

Lots of people who've spent much of their lives trying to attain a certain level of physical or emotional satisfaction feel short-changed for, all too often, they find that what they've worked so hard to achieve has not brought them the internal satisfaction they've been looking for. Sometimes, it manifests itself as the need to down size and simplify. So instead of maintaining a house designed to take care of a family during those growing up years, some people sell these homes, or businesses or farms, and move to a living situation that requires less upkeep.

"Here I am eighty and I'm free ... I can play however I want to."
– Ann St. John Hawley

However you bring it about, create the reality you'd like to see. Child rearing, careers, professions or work life may be done or near done, and this time can be very liberating. It can provide new avenues to explore, expand horizons and provide opportunities to give to family and friends in a way that's different from when we were younger. That was a time of carrying a full load of responsibilities. Now, we have more time to be more responsible to ourselves. In simplifying, we make space for new things in the mind, opening up new ways of thinking and being. A peaceful mind, one that knows how to achieve that place of a mind at rest, can make the space for a different kind of "knowing" to enter.

Chapter Three
Focus on Change

*W*hatever it is we decide to do and explore, we shouldn't be afraid of change – it's the way of the Universe. As the famous Danish philosopher Kierkegaard said, "Without risk there is no faith." We can also see that without change there is no growth. Sometimes as we get older we become more entrenched in what we're doing and more attached to that which we know. It often doesn't seem worthwhile to make any effort to bring about change, and frequently we find ourselves resisting it when it presents itself. We might think we no longer have what it takes or we're unable to justify it on whatever grounds we choose to use as measures of judgment. Often, we simply don't have enough faith in ourselves to create the challenge but meeting it once we've created it might be easier than we think.

Creating challenge, or just recognizing the freedom in the choices we have in front of us is

"I like discovering new things."

– ANN ST. JOHN HAWLEY

"I honestly think the change has kept me younger ... because I'm not in a competitive world as I used to be."

– HELEN ABRAMOWITZ

"The first half of life is just a preparation for the second half."

"When I became seventy I said life begins at seventy because I really felt like I knew where I was going."
— TED EGRI

empowering. It encourages us to become more open and allows the space for things, other than those that are known and familiar, to enter into our consciousness. So instead of feeling that we've already accomplished a good deal of what we think we've had to, we may realize that might only be a foundation on which to build. We may still have almost another half of our lives to go! Let's ensure that we provide for ourselves not only the quality of life now while we can still enjoy it, but help provide the quality of life we'd like to see ourselves enjoying in our later years. These years of mid-life can be some of the most rewarding in our lives. They can also help prepare the way for our future. One of the ways we can ensure that is to be aware, right now, of how to best take care of ourselves so that later on, ideally, others won't have to do that for us.

There are no guarantees that all that we may do for ourselves now to build and maintain a healthy state of well-being, physically, mentally and spiritually, will ensure the quality of life that we envision in those later years. But why not prepare ourselves in the very best ways we know how? Meanwhile we can achieve the gratification that these changes can bring us now.

Being able to transform a middle aged body that seems to have succumbed to the laws of gravity, where all your muscles may feel like they're falling, into one that is fit and toned can give you the confidence you might need to show you what positive changes you can achieve. The body is truly astounding in its ability to heal itself, to submit to healthy changes, like weight loss if needed, or stronger muscles and firmer flesh. When you find your endurance increasing, your flexibility enhanced, your strength and stamina returning, you'll also recognize that you were the one to bring about those changes and manifest the reality you wanted to see. It may not always be easy, but a strong positive attitude, a good measure of discipline and dedication and the willingness to do whatever it takes to bring about the desired results are all the tools you need.

"I am totally able to be responsible to myself."

"I work at being independent, in being healthy."

– HELEN ABRAMOWITZ

The mind is quite amazing, too, in its ability to be flexible. Programming can be changed or modified. We're now in a place where we can think more independently and be much less concerned with the judgments of others. Our thoughts, after all, are uniquely our own and an expanding mind allows for all kinds of possibilities to make themselves known. R.D. Laing, the ground breaking Scottish psychiatrist, once said, "Freedom is an explosion of possibilities." That can be a pretty exhilarating concept at this stage of our lives. We don't want to ever waste our time on "should haves" like, " I should have studied a foreign language, traveled more, become a poet, raised orchids, been a carpenter, gotten more education, worked harder, worked less!" There's plenty of time (we hope) to do those things without looking back on what has already transpired. We also don't need to look forward to the results as much as we might have during a previous time in our lives.

"I don't know what's happening, I don't know where it's leading to, but I'm more and more excited about what I'm going to do next – that's the fun part of it, I don't know what's going to happen next and I look forward to finding out!"

– TED EGRI

If you like the idea of traveling and don't have the financial resources to give you a couple of months in Europe, Africa, South America, or India, maybe buying a used camper and hitting the road in your own country could give you all that you want or need to do. Discovering other places, landscapes, and exchanges with different people can take place with very little more than simply the incentive to make it happen. It's the same with whatever other change we want to see and experience. If we're in reasonably good health and of sound minds and open hearts, we can open new vistas within and outside of ourselves.

Challenging our minds as well as our bodies can bring exciting results. Problem solving can be a lot easier now with a perspective that can draw upon past experiences. New decisions can be made from a mind that is less stressed out with anxiety about the outcome. A shift of perspective from one that was rooted in a view of controlling to one of allowing things to reveal themselves provides room for completely new situations to present themselves. The taking on of new projects or new relationships can provide a sense of satisfaction and fulfillment and sometimes awe at what is "out there" for us.

Once we can clear the mind and let go of extraneous "stuff," we'll find a lot more space has opened for new things to enter, for new thoughts and ideas to unfold. It should be a lot easier now to release some of those things that often cluttered the mind, like anxiety and worry, insecurity and excessive planning of our agendas, daily or long-range. What a lot of time and energy is now freed up when we can rid ourselves of mind "clutter." Much of what we have in our minds is extraneous anyway, and I think we come to a realization that we can be a lot more comfortable with less, and that means thinking as well as material things.

It seems that we're now more concerned about dealing with what is on hand, rather than with future projections or expectations or

"Thoughts are things, so be careful of what you collect or what you think because you're going to collect a lot of garbage."

"If things are sitting around taking up space, put it in storage."

– DALE AMBURN

dwelling on past history. The latter can really be an energy rip-off, since the past is already done and the only thing we can do about it is to learn from it. Isn't that the real purpose of all our experiences? So if we focus on the past to see our mistakes and then go about trying to balance some of the fallout from them, that can be a positive activity. If we look at the past with regret and it helps us make the determination to take a different path that, too, can be positive. But if we view our past by dwelling on injustices that have been visited upon us, by losses we were not able to control and not go on from there, then it's like throwing good money after bad. We're simply feeding a bad situation with more energy, which is only a further waste.

It is healthier, by far, to concentrate on "being in the moment" which means being more fully present and paying attention to what's happening now. It should be a lot easier to do this, because for most of us, there is less to distract us now. I say most of us because I'm fully aware that during these mid-years we've taken on different responsibilities, like the care of elderly parents who might be in poor health, or if not being completely responsible for providing this care, we might have to be involved in making difficult decisions as to how that care will be provided. We may still be involved in paying off mortgages and other loans with decreased incomes, or helping our kids with their needs, without ade-quate resources.

However, problems are part of life, and if we've learned nothing else from these years of living in the world, we no doubt understand this. Problems get solved, one way or another, but how we handle problems is really the mark of maturity. Getting stressed out does nothing but affect both ourselves and others adversely. If, instead, we can act with compassion and from a place of integrity, free of manipu-lation, and a faith in the ongoing process we call life, we stand a far better chance of solving problems with a clearer mind and more open heart.

Section Two
Enhance the
Quality of Your Life

A series of systems

Functioning independently

All interconnected

Chapter Four
Exercise

*A*lthough there's an implied agreement that this book would give no answers, quote no other books or authorities, physical, mental or spiritual – not even contain a bibliography (no less footnotes or references), there are certain actions I consider to be necessary to ensure the state of well-being we are striving to achieve. For starters, I feel it's imperative to incorporate a program of physical fitness. The program, however, must be your own. What we do at this juncture requires that we chart a routine that works for us. I believe it's our responsibility to take charge of that which is our own domain, our body, and keep it strong and healthy, functioning at its best.

There are many wonderful books that can guide us with exercise programs that are designed to keep our bodies fit and healthy. (Anyone who is still breathing and conscious has glimpsed many of the health, diet, food and recipe books that are on the shelves of

"You've got to keep the parts working,"
– BILL STALLCUP

"If you don't want to let it get you down all the time, you have to work through it."
– PAT STALLCUP

bookstores, nutrition centers, natural health food and super markets. Many of these authors have built their foundation upon years of working with clients and patients in specific programs). There is no lack of material available, and choosing that which may help in determining a program specifically for you could provide a reading opportunity that is both stimulating and inspiring. It might seem a little daunting at first, but in the end it will be you who will make the decision about a program that best fits your particular needs. Some might be effective, while others simply might not work for you. There may be a little bit of trial and error to determine which ones might contribute to your ultimate goal which is a firm commitment to an exercise routine, but that's part of the process.

It's easiest to start out on the physical, as that's the most apparent place to focus. By now, most of us have recognized that not only has our eyesight changed, but that, most definitely, our metabolism has slowed down and our ability to process the fueling of our bodies requires a little extra help, sometimes a jump start.

Exercise is obviously of critical importance in keeping physically fit. Luckily, it's available to everyone and is completely free, (unless you make specific choices that do involve a cash investment, but the returns can be enormous). However you choose to design your program, your goal is to get into shape, to become and stay fit. There are many books, tapes and videos describing ways of doing this. There can be recommendations by friends who've found something of help to them. It might feel intimidating or overwhelming to decide or formulate your own program, but the key is to begin. Don't postpone, or think about how or where to start. Just start somewhere. No matter how out of shape you are, or how much you've become resigned to it, this is an exciting time to start a lifelong commitment to an exer-

"Dance is my favorite form of exercise."

- ANN ST. JOHN HAWLEY

cise program, and by so doing, a life long commitment to a strong and sound body.

One easy way for a lot of people to get started is to join a gym or health club. Sometimes that's just enough structure to get you involved, either through classes or by working out with a personal trainer until you get enough confidence to do it on your own. Often, a spa or health club will offer special programs for "senior citizens." It's a comfortable way to begin, and you don't have to be intimidated by strong, buff young bodies that are already toned. You can also work easily at your own pace, anywhere from keeping up with the thirty-five year old instructor, or just taking it easy, until you develop those muscles to the point where they respond without protest. There's also a socialization that takes place at a fitness center that may appeal to you. For many, it becomes a support group where everyone is in more or less the same situation and genuinely applauds the positive changes that take place in their friends. For those who feel self conscious, or don't really like engaging in those kinds of activities in the company of others, there are lots of other alternatives.

"After a friend suggested that I join the spa, I became hooked."

– Helen Abramowitz

You can easily work out at home, either alone or with friends. Why not sample some of the videos, tapes and books, designed for aerobic activity with emphasis on cardio vascular exercises, as well as strengthening and toning the body? All you have to do is find one that works for you. Once you start seeing the benefits and feeling the results of what renewed energy will do for your mind, body and spirit, it will be like crossing a threshold. You'll find yourself looking forward to "working out" rather than thinking of it as "work you should do." And when you find yourself experiencing time periods when you're not consciously involved in an exercise program, you might be surprised at how deprived you feel and look forward to getting going again.

Tom Morrow, who's been in the same exercise classes as the ones I attend is an outstanding example of someone who works out with the vigor and enthusiasm of an instructor half his age. He says "I really feel bad if I miss classes, especially if I can't go for a full week. I like to go three to four times a week."

Sometimes we put exercise off indefinitely, and sometimes we feel that it might be too late to begin. Certain events may trigger our need to initiate what we already know is a good and necessary thing, but have postponed doing for various reasons. We are often jolted into the necessity of changing our way of life through disease or illness, which is an overt sign of imbalance in our bodies. It is far better to start off with a sound exercise program before we experience the consequences of disease or illness that maybe could have been averted.

For years I put off consciously exercising with various rationalizations. For one thing (I told myself), I did a lot of physical activity as part of my daily work in the hand woven textile business, carrying, pulling, folding, and unfolding rugs. It seemed that I walked miles every day from one part of my gallery to another. I also felt as strong as I ever did and had myself convinced that was true. My energy level, always high, remained the same. So far, so good. My need for an exercise program never presented itself in a glaring way.

Except, perhaps, that I was overweight. But that, too, was subtle. I had always been small and still thought of myself that way, although my clothes had changed a size or two. And I wore looser clothing like ethnic huipiles that hid a multitude of flaws. Although I could hardly be called fat, I was no longer petite in spite of my reluctance to admit it. I knew that getting back into shape would be harder past fifty, but I kept putting it off. Of course I also felt I didn't have the time and being the way I was seemed perfectly acceptable.

For me, making the first move in joining a spa was not the result of a specific event or "wake up" call. I still felt a young fifty-five but I finally realized it was time to do something and I knew that could be the place to find out whether or not that would work for me. When I first started going, I had no idea of where to begin. I started slowly by joining a water aerobics class, which I thought would be low impact, but found it just didn't seem to be enough for me. Then I started a couple of other classes, testing what felt right for me. At first I found a "step" class more challenging than I had realized it would be, which was my first clue as to how out of shape I actually was.

I decided to ask the instructor to be my personal trainer. As well as continuing with aerobics classes, I now received instruction in cardio vascular activities, which included treadmill, rowing, stationery bicycle and step machines. At the same time I was lifting weights, starting with light weights and gradually increasing weight and repetitions as I became stronger and my endurance improved. After a while I got some help with diet specifically aimed at moderate weight loss, and lowering of body fat level. The discipline was just what I needed.

Within a couple of years I found my muscle tone improved, my endurance noticeably increased and enough of a weight loss to be detected in the way my clothes fit, especially in the waistline. There was also a decrease in my ratio of body fat, definitely healthier. Most importantly, exercise was now part of my life. How significant all of this was to my general state of well-being was demonstrated when I suddenly found myself one summer day unable to stand from an acute attack of abdominal pain which didn't abate. The next day found me in the emergency room of the hospital, hooked up to various machines, undergoing a battery of tests while the surgeon evaluated my condition. It was apparent that there was an intestinal blockage, since my digestive system was completely closed down, but what was causing it was unknown. After being fed through an IV for more than a week with no change whatsoever, I agreed with the surgeon that he should go ahead with exploratory surgery and deal with whatever was causing the condition.

Fortunately, the operation was taken care of quickly and easily with no anxiety or stress. I was home a few days later, my six-inch cut held together with staples and tape under a neat bandage. The initial stage of recovery was without complications and my energy started returning within a few months. Six months later, I felt as good as new and started thinking about a gradual reintroduction of exercise. Obviously, I was grateful for the positive way my body responded and was convinced that the work I had done the previous couple of years, which had included a good exercise program as well as a regime of daily supplements, contributed to the speedy recovery.

When I did once again resume an active exercise program I found myself strong and fit, with the only evidence of my medical encounter a slightly lopsided (I like to think of it as somewhat charming) vertical scar. I have several friends with their own brands of scars and surgical experiences, who share in a similar lifestyle of attention to their bodies, their minds and their spirits. They look and feel great! No one knows when they're going to find themselves in these kinds of emergency situations, but being prepared on all levels helps significantly in how we experience them.

A consistent routine of exercise not only provides better muscle tone, strength and increased bone density, but results in better flexibility, increasingly important as we get older, so that we're less likely to suffer from pulled muscles. As we see our strength and endurance increase, we are reminded of the good we're accomplishing for ourselves. At first, we may huff and puff as we walk up a hill, but how nice it is, a few months later, to be able to do the same walk, breathing with no strain and maybe being able to carry on a conversation at the same time! We may have started out with 2 lb. weights with four repetitions and now may have tripled that. Again, it's not always how far we've got-ten, but continuing. Accept with satisfaction what you've achieved, but do what it takes to maintain. Starting and stopping for periods of time doesn't really do much in keeping the body fit as a way of life.

"Early on, I developed high blood pressure ... the cardio vascular activity is really important to me."

"I know if I quit, I'll go downhill."

– BILL STALLCUP

Always listen to your body. The more attuned you are, the more quickly you will feel what the right rhythm is for you. If you're pushing too hard you'll realize it and if you strain muscles, you'll know to take it easy. Sports injuries are very common, and if you feel twinges of pain, or if you've thrown something out of alignment, ease up and get some help before it becomes a problem. I find that taking long, hot showers after I've exercised helps keep my muscles from tightening up. I've come to love the ladies' locker room and enjoy tak-ing the time to relax after a good workout.

Although I believe that everyone should develop their own exercise routine, there are certain things that will help in any program. Every workout should start out with a warm-up, whether it's in the weight room, the aerobics room or the room where fitness classes are held, in a health club or your own living room. That helps loosen up your muscles so that they're better able to follow the demands made upon them. Likewise, every workout should end up with stretching, which releases the muscles and alleviates strain on the worked areas. It's also a superb way to relax and get into a quiet space after the active one.

Balance should be practiced as part of an exercise routine and that can take place anywhere at any time. Standing on one leg (arms out for balance if necessary, or even holding on to something to begin with), and looking in various directions is a nice challenge. Perhaps when we were younger, balance wasn't an issue, but like so many other things, it becomes something to be more aware of as we grow older.

Stretching regularly as part of that routine will keep your body flexible and will help avoid extra strain on all those body parts, like muscles and joints. Breathing properly is also an imperative and should be incorporated, consciously, with every exercise movement. Don't hold in the breath, but breathe in and breathe out with awareness – and rhythmically. Use proper form to avoid injuries. A personal trainer or aerobics instructor can really help with this. Just going through the motions isn't enough, and knowing and using the proper form has nothing to do with "looking good," but "doing good" for your body. Most importantly, it will reduce the risk of injuries, which sometime occur when improper form is used, placing unnecessary stress and strain on the body.

Keeping limber and flexible is extremely important for our bodies at any time, but especially as we get older. Although some of us may still think we can do what we did twenty years ago (and some of us actually can), for most of us our strength, endurance and muscle tone has diminished. Exercise certainly helps and the results can be amazing even if you've not consciously exercised since high school or college. The body is quite resilient, and conscious exercise can do wonders in restoring and renewing a body that all too many of us have taken for granted.

Aerobic exercise is only one way to go. There are a lot of other options, including yoga, tai chi, chi gong, stretching and multiple combinations of activities. Any of these disciplines can be very effective in releasing tensions stored up in the body and can provide a better sense of well-being, of the mind as well as the body. These are ancient techniques that have proved effective over the ages, and have been used by literally millions of people. It is a thing of joy to see a master of these disciplines move with ease and grace and fluidity through a series of movements specifically designed to enhance our feeling of well-being. And it's inspiring to see that many of these masters are well over the age of fifty!

Back in the old days, in our societies and still in many rural based societies, walking was a way of life. It was how you got from here to there. Now, we walk consciously because of all the exercises, it's the one that affects all of our organs and muscles, providing aerobic activity that strengthens our heart, loosens up our muscles, expands our lungs and burns some calories at the very same time! And it's not only 100% free, but provides innumerable fringe benefits.

If you have the good fortune to live in an area where you are surrounded by a natural environment, it puts you back in touch with that. Sunrises, sunsets, the sound of birds, of running streams, the sight and smell of flowers, of trees, of the changing seasons enrich with their beauty. If you tune into the solitude of walking, it's a time away from outside distractions, no ringing of telephones, no blaring of other voices on the television, no demands on your attention. It's a time that's "all yours." Some of my best thinking (or respite from thoughts) takes place when I'm walking. It's also a time when we can exercise our consciousness by noting details like specific rocks on the side of the road, or certain children out playing at that particular time, how the temperature is changing, or the light.

And it's something we can do any place, any time, for as long as we want to, alone or with friends, in the city or in the country, in a familiar environment or when we're traveling. It takes very little effort (once you've gotten yourself in gear) and requires no equipment. Once you get into walking it, too, becomes part of your life style, and you won't want to give it up. Very often, when your body feels tight, walking helps warm up muscles and provides more flexibility. It's always important to have the attitude that you're doing something not because you have to, but because you want to. Very often, we've built in a resistance to a particular activity, and some people view walking as a chore. If this is the case, an intentional shift in attitude will do wonders. You might find yourself very pleased by how much you appreciate having incorporated walking into your daily life.

With walking, as with any form of exercise, the key is "staying with it." This can happen most easily if it becomes something you enjoy doing. When starting out, keep in mind to work at whatever level is comfortable. Challenging yourself at the beginning might prove to be more of a detriment than a benefit, for you might find yourself getting discouraged. But if you start slowly and have no expectations, you'll soon discover your own comfort level, and can move on from there with increased time and accelerated pace. If there's too much demand, your body will let you know. If there's not enough, you'll naturally find yourself wanting to work harder, walk faster or longer until you get to the level you feel is right for you.

Some years ago I joined a friend on his daily "hike." Since he had just had surgery a few weeks earlier, he cut his hike down to three miles. But for the last twenty-five years or more, he's been doing his morning hike of five miles most days. We live in the mountains and while half the year is absolutely beautiful, the other half during the winter can be challenging with lots of snow and temperatures below zero for long periods of time. For Jim, it's all the same – all of it's beautiful! It's just a question of which particular boots he wears, or which jacket, hat and gloves. Hiking not only keeps his body toned and in superb shape, but keeps him in touch with the changes in the trees, the skies, and with himself. It's not only "part of his program," it's what he's incorporated into his life, just as much as eating and sleeping.

Whatever it is that you decide to do, you must maintain. It's not a question of getting to a particular point and concluding that you're "there" (even if you think you look like you did twenty years ago and feel as strong as you did then too). Exercise is a life long commitment and not simply a means to an end. A strong body is not the only thing we must concern ourselves with, but it's an important part of the equation in keeping fit and healthy, headed toward the next fifty years in as good shape as we can provide, by paying attention to our bodies now.

Chapter Five
Health and Food

*H*ere in our affluent society where so many people are preoccupied with their appearance, the call to shed excess weight provides a major market. It is quite a statement to make when we consider that one of the major problems that exist for most of the world is getting enough to eat, simply to survive. But in our society, along with both the quantity and diversity of foods available to us, we seem to suffer from an excess of eating, resulting in a constant striving to lose weight. Unfortunately, this excessive consuming of food is not our only problem. Much of our population eats food that not only is not good for them but can actually be injurious to their health and well-being. And we are bombarded with propaganda from the time we are children to consume food that has little if any nutritional value.

If you find it useful to have a couple of books or magazine articles around to remind you of what's nutritionally sound, and what the calorie count is of specific foods, or what combinations are most effective, that's great, and even better if you stay on top of it at all times by paying proper attention to what you eat. Sometimes it helps to use visualizations. I like to think of the various enzymes snapping to attention every time a new shipment of food arrives to enter the digestive system. Sometimes I hear them groaning, "Oh, what is she doing to us this time?" or "here we go again, it's another day of hard labor!" I picture them as being content when I send down something nourishing and easy to digest.

We do not have to have a college degree in nutrition to know what's good for us. There are certain foods that we should eliminate whenever possible, for there is simply nothing nutritious about them, and they can definitely affect our bodies in adverse ways. The most obvious foods to avoid are those that are laced with chemicals whose effects, unfortunately, do not necessarily come to an end when the wastes are disposed of, but lodge in the cells of our bodies where they may establish long-term residual traces. High on the list of foods to avoid also are refined foods. First the nutrients are removed in the processing and then supplements are added later on, which never actually replace that which has been removed in the first place. Now we're dealing with both supplemental (in the form of "reinforced" vitamins and minerals) and chemical additives as well.

Fast foods impact upon the environment as well as on our bodies in any number of ways. To begin with, huge areas of rain forests are cut down daily to provide more and more pasture land on which to graze the animals that are later processed to serve the millions of hamburgers that have become a way of life, now world wide. These rain forests are a tremendous and critical source of oxygen for the entire planet, absorbing carbon monoxide and giving off oxygen. What an incredible system, if we don't tamper with it!

Another thing to be aware of concerning the food that is served through fast food chains, is the use of chemicals and preservatives that are added at every stage, from the food consumed by the cattle, to that which is added to prevent spoilage during the vast distance of delivery to the final consumption of that "tasty" burger. The ill effects are further compounded by the use of grease and oil used to prepare both it and its favorite accompaniment, french fries. We have been programmed to accept this way of cooking as tasty and appealing. But what does it actually do to us, besides providing a "quick fix" food-wise? It is a great market geared toward those of us involved in a fast paced society, where time is of the essence, and many feel they simply don't have that time to shop for fresh ingredients, prepare the food, serve it, linger to savor it and then clean up. Sometimes just the energy of simply thinking about what to prepare is too much, and fast foods seem to be so convenient!

In a society that is so accelerated, the whole concept of eating leisurely and enjoying the preparation of food that requires time and patience is quickly disappearing. Rather than doing things for the pleasure they bring, we find ourselves victims of that "have to" imperative. Now it's the rare person who doesn't have lists of what they "have to" take care of, with all the attenuating feelings of anxiety, stress, tension and guilt that often accompany the doing, rather than taking care of things as best we can. It often feels that we have these impossible goals to fulfill, just to get through daily activities. Being on "overwhelm" provides a fertile ground to indulge in these "quick fixes" in spite of the fact that we might know better.

According to some research, there is far less obesity in countries like Italy, where the taking of a meal is an important aesthetic experience, savored slowly, than in

"All foods are a gift of God – don't ever eat with a negative mind set."

"We live in a society of illnesses of lifestyle and mind set ... we're not dying from diphtheria, smallpox and plague. We're dying from mind set and illnesses of lifestyle. The former goes out, says, 'I have to go pick apricots this afternoon,' the latter says, 'I'm going to pick apricots this afternoon because they're ready.'"

– DALE AMBURN

the United States. In many cultures it is a time for the family to get together sharing not only the food, but conversation concerning their personal experiences, thoughts and feelings.

Food is not only what we must have to fuel our systems but can be a celebration, if we shift our perspective. In the weaving village where I have been working for more than twenty-five years, the invitation to share "comida" with families is a special one. It not only is a break in "doing business," but a time of relaxing, of exchanging conversation and catching up on what's taken place in our lives, as well as the appreciation of the food that's been prepared with great care. The Zapotec custom of thanking their guests first for being there is not only a reflection of their graciousness, but an appreciation of being together in the sharing of the meal.

One of the rewards that comes from preparing your own food is that you know what goes into it, unlike buying prepared foods where often "ignorance is bliss." For that reason, I recommend strongly that you eat organically whenever you have the choice. It's important that we avoid the intake of chemicals whenever we can, pesticides and herbicides being right up the on the chart of what not to take into our systems. Now, with chemically engineered foods being treated with those toxic materials, some grains reach maturation with the toxic treatment built in from the time of their inception.

Read labels, not only for the amount of calories, but the ingredients as well, to determine the kind of sugars used and their use or lack of use of chemicals. Be conscious, be aware! Although we are now referring specifically to food, it's the way we must live our lives, especially at this stage when we want to give our bodies all the

"I live mostly on fruits and vegetables – I remain healthy and have a healthy life style. Each morning I take a walk, a very long walk. I eat organic foods as much as I can – I enjoy them. It feels good to eat well. I don't have alcohol, coffee, or fried foods."

– TED EGRI

help we can in maintaining healthy balances, well functioning systems, and organs that do not have to suffer inordinate
strains.

Be careful about high calorie snacks. Many of these are
presented as "healthy," but upon scrutiny, we often discover
a high content of sugar or saturated fats. Figure out when
you're most susceptible to consuming food you know is not
particularly good for you, and try to find a healthy substitute. If you eat a little more lightly, stopping before you have
that feeling of being "full," you'll reduce your stomach's
expectation of what it's accustomed to receiving in order to
be satisfied. Cutting down is not cutting out, and there is
often just as much to be realized from smaller amounts more
frequently, rather than waiting until you get to that point of
feeling hunger deprivation. Healthy late night snacks can
often be a challenge to the imagination, but you can find a
healthy substitute there as well. Sometimes something as
simple as a cup of herbal tea can do the trick. If you feel
completely unsatisfied unless you have something more sub-
stantial, try having just a little; you will eventually get to the
point where you don't expect so much anymore.

If you're unsure about what foods are good for you or
overwhelmed by your choices of recommended "diets," you
should be working with a doctor or health care provider to
plan a working food program that is satisfying to you and
provides you with the health benefits needed. Just as in exercise, working with an instructor or personal trainer to teach
you the proper program and the way it should be used most
effectively and safely, a doctor, nutritionist or health care
provider can give you the information you need to work out
a healthy way of approaching eating. Keep in mind however,
that many western doctors recommend processed diet foods,
so you might want to investigate the kind of professional with
an inclination toward natural foods. Fortunately there are
more and more doctors, including those who practice alter-

native treatments, who are approaching medicine in a more holistic way and integrate their suggestions for healthy diet as part of a preventative program as well as treatment for specific disorders. Again, eating consciously is not simply for weight loss but, like exercise, should become a way of life.

There is no need to "reward" yourself with food. The reward is in knowing you're doing something positive for yourself, not only to prolong your life, but to provide for a better quality of life down the line as well as now. There are many alternatives on the market that are healthy substitutes to what you may be used to and find hard to give up. You just have to make the switch. Instead of a diet that's heavy in meat, especially red meat and pork, you might (if you haven't already) put more emphasis on fish or fowl. You might discover that you're just as happy. Discover tofu, tempeh, soy and vegetable burgers. Textured vegetable protein can be extremely versatile.

Eating out can still be fun if it's done consciously. Find out from the waitperson how a particular food is prepared, what's in the sauce or soup. There's such a variety to choose from on most menus that it shouldn't be difficult to find something that is not only enjoyable, but healthy as well. So much of eating out is built around socialization that the food is only a part of the experience. Good food doesn't have to mean high calories, but well prepared with ingredients that are good for us as well as pleasing to the palate.

Drinking plenty of water should be part of everyone's daily routine and you'll find having water with meals instead of soda, beer, soft drinks, or even fruit juices can become the expected accompaniment. Just having a glass of water along with something light can sometimes work for those times in between meals as well, when we feel the need for "something." You don't necessarily have to be thirsty to consume a little extra water.

An intensive focus on what we eat can easily become

excessive and somewhat irritating to people around us, when we go on and on reporting every morsel we consume (or don't). It's a lot more fun at family gatherings, for example, to simply avoid the things we feel we should without talking about it, and just take a little of those things we might like to have, without having to splurge and go overboard. It can be nice to have a piece of birthday cake to celebrate, but a small slice can be just as satisfying as an oversized one, once we establish the mind set. Sometimes we just feel like a "splurge" for no reason whatsoever. As long as we don't fall into the "one thing leads to another" syndrome, we should be able to control ourselves when we feel like splurging, as long as it's done mindfully. If you're going to do this on occasion, you might as well enjoy it, without those horrendous feelings of guilt, which have no place whatsoever. We are, after all, responsible for our own decisions and shouldn't have to frag-ment ourselves into degenerate "indulgers" or rigorous "policers." Having an occasional cookie or two (my choice), or whatever you might consider your particular indulgence is really not going to make any difference to the person who has a good grasp on what they consider to be the desired way of eating healthily.

If we just stay conscious and aware, we can enjoy life and still maintain a healthy way of living. One would hope that a responsible adult could take charge of what they know to be good for them. There is such an incredible amount of infor-mation available that we need to discriminate and determine what works for us. It's really not a one-size-fits-all approach, as if a particular way or plan or formula is the only one. It may work for some, but it may not be the most effective plan for us. Just as in exercise, develop your own program. It's no secret which foods are best for us, and in what quantity. Reading health and nutrition magazines, rather than ones that emphasize special "diets" will probably be more helpful in the long run because the articles do not focus on the "quick fix" or immediate gratification of diets that are hard to maintain. Rather, they are designed to be more informative concerning the positive properties of particular foods and may provide new information about the beneficial aspects of specific vitamins, minerals and natural herbs, and the way they act on the body's chemistry.

Like many others, I have found that bringing the "wrong" kind of food into the house, thinking we'll indulge in moderation and only on occasion, doesn't always work that way. If it's there, it somehow gets eaten and the temptation always beckons (unless we've developed a strong discipline). So, at this point, the preference is simply not to have in the house the things I know we're best off without. If I feel that I'd like to have something special when I'm outside my home, as in a restaurant or having dinner with friends or family, that's much easier. As in every thing we do, staying conscious should always be our guide. Our bodies are generally pretty good about letting us know what foods are and aren't good for us. Stay in touch!

Chapter Six
Those Addictive Foods and Substances

*V*ery few of us are blissfully ignorant of what's good and not good for us. It would be hard to live in the world and be unaware that we should not use tobacco. We not only harm ourselves when we do, but others around us who are innocent bystanders and not the least bit interested in coating their lungs with the noxious waste. This is especially hard on babies and small children whose respiratory systems are particularly vulnerable. And, as is true in so many cases, they have nothing to say about it, but are victimized by it. Although for many years the tobacco industry has steadily maintained that smoking was not injurious to health, it has been proven otherwise and "second hand" smoking is almost as bad. In spite of all the information we now have on the injurious affects of smoking, many young people are already addicted. Since the addictive substances have been increased, it makes it more difficult than ever to stop. But, with the same information, many people fifty or over have consciously chosen to stop a habit they may have had for the majority of their adult lives, not an easy thing to do for anyone who has become addicted to a substance.

Alcohol can so often be abused and affect many others in a deleterious manner that it should be used only in moderation. As tobacco has its place in ceremonials performed by Native American peoples, so alcohol, too, might have its place when its use does not become excessive. But when it's abused, the harmful effect on vital organs such as the liver can result in premature death, or certainly complications of existing health conditions. Since it converts to sugar, it can also raise blood sugar levels unnecessarily, causing other health problems.

The effects on others caused by alcohol abuse and its impact on families, as well as society in general, go far beyond the individual who abuses alcohol making it, in all too many cases, deadly. The statistics for alcohol related deaths resulting from drivers under the influence is overwhelming and after many years the organization known as MADD (Mothers Against Drunk Driving) has been influential in getting many local laws changed to acknowledge this crime, and then seeing that they are enforced. Abuse of women and children can often be associated with excessive use of alcohol, as well as the loss of jobs and homes. The results of stress, tension and anxiety created by alcoholic behavior impact not only in the short term, but frequently have long-term damaging effects, thus influencing the next generation as well. Many people well into adulthood are actively working on the deep-rooted and negative psychological affects of a childhood in an alcoholic family.

Every book or magazine article that I've read that seems sensible usually eliminates the intake of caffeine, except in small amounts. That means coffee, non-herbal teas and soft drinks such as colas, the last of which are further exacerbated by being carbonated.

Oils and grease, especially those that are used in fried foods (another no), should be minimized, particularly saturated fats, which are hard to digest. Investigate which oils, such as olive oil, are the best to use. There are foods that contain the "good" fats, such as those with omega 3 fatty acids, but generally one should maintain a high consciousness regarding the intake of fats and grease, for not only do they add weight, but are a challenge to our intestinal system which we like to keep in as good working order as possible. It's easy enough, if one is controlling their food consumption, to simply eliminate saturated fats as much as possible, which includes the intake of fried foods.

When we talk about sugars and sweeteners, many people think if they just use artificial sweeteners it's perfectly okay. Well, it's not. Whatever their base, natural or chemical, the body reads it as sugar. But the artificial sweeteners that are chemically derived cannot possibly do us any good. It's practically impossible to know all the ingredients that have been put into foods unless we prepare it ourselves, and many that seem to be a healthy choice are actually high in sugars of various kinds. That's why reading labels is so important. It is particularly difficult for me to talk about sugar intake because, like so many people, I've been somewhat addicted, and still have a hard time resisting my favorite chocolate chip cookie. (I've done pretty well on eliminating ice cream, which has the double whammy effect of sugar and butter fat in addition to various and sundry additives).

I think a great aid is the old adage of Socrates, "know thyself." The first part is recognition and acknowledgement that we have become addicted to certain things which can impair our health and well-being. Critical to any program dealing with addiction is this first step. The problem is that many of us will not admit to ourselves that there is an addictive pattern. "I just have to have my coffee," they say or "I don't feel a meal is complete without dessert." Maybe it's "my father smoked all his life and he lived until ninety-two." However, once we recognize that some of our patterns may be injurious to our health, we can set about trying to curb those tendencies, if not eliminate them. Once again, we can try looking for an alternative. Sometimes preparing something yourself that feels like a treat, but that will substitute honey or stevia for refined sugar, can satisfy your longings for something sweet. I've found that rather than just having a selection of fruit, cutting it up into salad and adding something special like berries, walnuts and/or yogurt makes it feel more like a special dessert.

If you've smoked or consumed alcohol for many years it might be that now is a much easier time of your life to quit, in spite of all the years you've done so. Some of the reasons you began in the first place may no longer be valid. Or maybe you're wiser now and don't particularly care what your peer group does. Perhaps you've learned that although some things might be difficult, the positive results you aim for are worth it. I'm sure we've all plowed through difficulties in our lives and have come to the realization that sometimes we simply have to make up our mind to take a particular course of action that might mean the saving of our job, our family or simply our life. It takes work, but like everything else we've discussed, we are rewarded with that sense of empowerment when we take charge of our lives by making conscious decisions.

Chapter Seven
Supplementing our Diet

*H*ealth magazines frequently focus on the latest develop-
ments in vitamins and supplements. This is another
area that can be completely overwhelming, especially with
"new studies" appearing almost constantly concerning the
various attributes of vitamins, minerals, naturopathic and
herbal remedies. It used to be if we were to take a good all
around daily vitamin and mineral supplement, we would think
that would be adequate. We know now that in addition to that,
there are specific vitamins and minerals that seem to have
good results for specific conditions and might help combat
the onslaught of certain diseases such as heart disease through
helping control high blood sugar or cholesterol levels.

If we were able to receive all the nutrients we need
from the food we eat we probably wouldn't even think
about supplements. But with soil depletion, environmental
pollution and the all-pervasive chemical residue in fruits and
vegetables as well as in meat, we simply don't receive the
high quality of food that was previously available to us.

Remember, the main premise of this book is not to provide any programs or suggestions except in the most general
way to promote a sound body, mind, and spirit. The way you

bring this about is distinctly your own. For that reason, I suggest nothing specific on this topic except that you do as much information gathering as possible to decide on supplements that work for you. It can vary also, until you find that you've achieved a general level of well-being and are not subject to contracting much in the way of passing colds, coughs, sore throats, flus or respiratory infections due to bacterial or viral attacks. This will let you know your immune system is functioning well and you must be doing something right.

The use of high quality supplements can be an important part of maintaining good health and taking naturally based supplements in place of chemically based ones is definitely preferable. If you're able to spend more on a high quality supplement, you'll no doubt get more in return, but always check it out, especially if you're dealing with a knowledgeable pharmacist, herbalist or nutritionist. Study carefully and discuss with these people what might be right for you. The key to maintaining the immune system at a high level requires continuity. If you are successful at warding off invasions of disease before they attack, the body will be able to take over and do its normal work. Prevention is much preferable to just dealing with symptoms and that can often be enhanced by a healthy balance of nutritional supplements. Whatever you do, be reasonable and be discriminating. Read labels carefully and check for side effects. Not everybody is the same and some people require less than more, in terms of dosage.

Anti-oxidants to help defend against free radicals can be useful in helping prevent the breakdown of the body's systems. There are attacks going on all the time on a molecular level and however we can help our systems of defense will go a long way in maintaining the desired state of good health. We're also working toward keeping ourselves from developing complications that might result in heart attacks, diabetes, and other breakdowns of our systems later in life.

Like so much of how we approach caring for ourselves, gathering information and then proceeding to take the supplements we feel we need can be aided by tuning into our own body and its specific needs. My body is a lot smaller and lighter than most bodies and I feel comfortable with a smaller dosage of whatever is recommended on the bottle. I also vary the supplements I take, although some are constant. Some times I skip several days. Whatever it is, it seems to work for me in keeping my immune system functioning properly with the aid of healthy food and conscious exercising. Although I'm reluctant to say it aloud or in print, the truth is I rarely get sick and have had years go by without having colds, sore throats, coughs or flus.

Common sense goes a long way in helping you determine which supplements to take. Many times when I pick up a new health magazine with articles discussing the studies made in regard to specific supplements, I file it away in the recesses of my mind. It doesn't seem like a good idea to experiment constantly with newly recommended supplements if what you're doing already works. Although I'm open to receive whatever information is out there, it seems a lot like trying every new lotion or potion that comes out on the market. There are all kinds of debates going on constantly about the positive effects of specific vitamins and minerals. Many require further study to determine what these effects are, or why one is preferred over another, or which combinations are most beneficial.

For thousands of years, people have been aware of healing effects of plants that were indigenous to their particular region of the world, and for many generations that information was passed on to the next one. Sometimes it worked, sometimes it didn't. If we were to get all that we need to maintain a healthy body, systems functioning at their maximum through a balanced and nutritious way of eating, we probably wouldn't need supplements. However, few of us receive all we need, no matter how we try to be conscious of what we eat, so if we can help maintain that immune system, treat specific imbalances or control high cholesterol or sugar levels through natural supplements rather than chemically based medications that often carry with them harmful side effects, it seems like a useful addition to our program of maintaining a healthy state of being.

Chapter eight
A Brief Look at Weight

*W*hy is there this often "obsessive" emphasis on weight loss and constant focus on how we look? It seems rather ironic that we are so preoccupied with this phenomenon while, at the same time, we're constantly bombarded with stimuli to consume food. It's hard to pick up any magazine without being enticed by sumptuous looking food presentations, complete with recipes, so that we can do more than just look and desire, but have the information about how to prepare it as well. And advertising, in all of its myriad forms, often focuses on food. Yet, much of our population is overweight.

Losing excess weight provides less of a strain on the heart and on all the vital organs, as well. Not only is the extra weight visible on the outside, but the same situation exists on the inside as well, with globs of fat surrounding those vital organs. Another exercise in visualization might help here too. Who needs it? It's excess baggage of the worst kind. Very few of us are the perfect anything, and on a physical level, where it is easiest to see, we must work with what we have. Not everyone is predisposed to look like those previously referred to magazine models, male or female. Some people have heavier frames, some more delicate, some can carry a little extra weight without it impairing their health and some (I'm told) will be forever thin.

When we address the intake of food in terms of weight loss, this becomes an issue many of us can relate to, whether we would like to drop a few extra pounds or are struggling with obesity. Unlike the weights at the spa, health club or home, which can be laid aside after use, some of us carry good deal of extra body weight day and night. This can seriously compromise our health. Losing weight simply to look good is the parallel to exercising so that we can look good. The purpose of keeping our bodies fit is not to look good, but to feel good. The looking good is like a bonus; it's a natural result of taking care of the body. With a toned body and a healthy diet, we'll naturally look better.

But what is "looking good?" Unfortunately, for much of our populace, especially women who are a prime target for the beauty and fitness market, looking good is synonymous with the images of magazine cover models. Although a good deal of this market is specifically aimed at women fifty and older, the models used are generally in their twenties. Well, no wonder they don't have wrinkles! Their bodies are firm and fit, and so can ours become, but let's face it, never again will they be as they were thirty years ago. A tree with a mature trunk and developed branches may not have the grace of a sapling, but it has its distinct form of beauty. A rose in full bloom, different from the promise of a rosebud, also has its distinct form of beauty. Maybe it's time to rethink how we view ourselves and what we consider as being beautiful!

"Every day you look the best you can, and that whatever happens, you work it out."

– Helen Abramowitz

Our aim in keeping ourselves fit is to regard our bodies with honor, and to be as good to them as they've been to us.

So in addition to exercising regularly, we need to be aware of eating properly and maintaining an acceptable weight level. This does not mean going out and buying every new book that comes out with still another incredible plan for weight loss. The formula we need to apply is a simple one: we burn up what we take in, using a balanced intake of nutritionally sound foods.

Whether you're on a weight loss program for the immediate goal of reducing your weight, or on a maintenance program, don't starve yourself. Your body will only read the lack of food as a temporary setback and start storing extra fat, until it gets to the point that it must use it. Meanwhile our minds read the situation as deprivation, which in turn frequently exaggerates the focus on food. Often, we develop perceived desires for sugar or carbohydrates, which turn into sugar. If you're working with a doctor or health care specialist, there may be a short-term program and a long-term program. But moderation goes a long way in maintaining a healthy food intake, and once you reach a comfort zone, you'll most likely want to stay there, just as when you see the results of incorporating a good exercise program.

For a good part of my adult life I took my body very much for granted, never dreaming that I, too, would approach that time of life where extra inches just accumulated. My weight was pretty constant according to my clothes and I never thought of owning a scale to check it out. With a change of years and lifestyle, the few pounds weight gain each year started to add up until there was a cumulative effect. When I finally did something about it and got rid of the extra weight, I found that I've achieved a pretty good and acceptable (to me) place, which is about five pounds more than my "low." I'm perfectly happy about the way I look, but more importantly, about the way I feel. When I find that I'm at the top of my "outside" parameter of what I consider optimum for me, I do something about it, like being more disciplined in those "extra indulgences" or cutting back a little on my quantity of food intake until I get back to where I feel is my comfort zone. Sometimes it includes a little extra "cardio" workout to burn off a few extra calories. That way I don't have to deal with the insidious "creeping up" that seems to affect us all.

There's no real mystery about how much we should weigh in order to maintain a healthy body. Obviously, this varies from person to person, but as in all the other fields of endeavor, we must be motivated by the desire to do what we can to maintain a healthy body, which means not putting excess strain on it. "Lightening our load" works positively on all levels and is the most obvious on a physical one.

Learn for yourself the weight you feel most comfortable at and do what you need to do to maintain that place. Some people find themselves needing to be extremely disciplined while others seem to be able to maintain by finding their own comfort zone, allowing themselves to indulge occasionally in certain situations knowing they simply will not let it get out of hand.

We not only accept our body, but by paying attention, we know we're honoring it by maintaining a sound level of good health. We know that to do this we must have, and continue to have as part of our life style, a sound exercise program and a healthy approach to food and supplements to maintain our immune system in good working order. We're doing this not to have a "beautiful" body, but a healthy one, which is a thing of beauty in itself. How many young people have you seen who are overweight and sloppy, smoke tobacco, overload on sugar and in general are not in good shape? Age really has nothing to do with fitness. When we are young we think we're indomitable. As we approach mid-life in our fifties, we realize that we have to become active participants in our own state of health by maintaining a balance where body, mind and spirit are integrated as a whole. When one part is out of balance, there's a need to bring it back into harmony.

Ideally, by this time in our lives, we will have learned to both honor and respect ourselves with the same love and compassion we extend to others. If we could quit expecting from ourselves something that someone is trying to sell us, like body image, and instead always keep in mind that a healthy body is a beautiful one we might be a lot more accepting of the way we look. Let's face it – we're not all made in the same image, nor do we come out of molds, with slight variations on the theme. I see it all as packaging, and how we look is simply the "wrapping" for what's within.

If we continue to focus on the external or the "wrapping" we will be constantly reinforcing the delusional image of "forever young." If we accept ourselves for who we are and honor the age we are right now, we will be making a different kind of statement. The kind of statement that says "I'm in pretty good shape considering that I'm 57, 67, 77 (or whatever)." Or, "I've got lines in my face – for those who can see, these are my stories." Yes, " my hair is getting gray – that must mean I'm on my way toward becoming an "elder." I would so much prefer to look the best I can

> *"Age is only a number, really."*
> – HELEN ABRAMOWITZ

at my authentic age than try to represent myself as ten or fifteen years younger, simply because there's been a conspiracy afoot to try to look as young as you can. How about, try to be as healthy as you can!

Section Three
A Matter of Mind

Unseen, unknown vibrations

About and around us

Those that resonate are our truths

Those that are presented to us

Might not be

Chapter Nine
Personal Growth

*A*s we address both exercise and food, we also engage our state of mind. Simply getting involved in a healthy balance of nutritious healthy food and an exercise program that keeps our bodies toned, our hearts strong, our strength and endurance levels up and our immune system maximized, indicates that we've already opted to make a firm commitment as to how we're going to live our lives. Rather than continue with old habits we know to be harmful to us, we've decided to live consciously.

Being aware on the physical level of the importance of beginning and maintaining an on-going fitness program that requires long term commitment and by keeping a positive attitude about why we're involved in our own program, enables us to see how this can now become our natural state of being. That's why we can never grow complacent when we achieve a particular goal, and

"Don't ask the questions unless you're ready to receive the responsibility that accompanies the answer - accountability - you can't plead ignorance when you know."

- DALE AMBURN

say, "I'm there!" We may be there for the moment, but it takes discipline, awareness and consciousness to stay "there." It's not an end, but a process, and the process works if we pay attention. This is a life long commitment and by getting one part of it in place, we become more aware of the other parts. We see how successful we can become in taking charge of our own lives in a healthy and happy way.

Personal growth is part of an ongoing process. With so much already behind us, such as careers, work and family obligations to which we have devoted so much time, energy and attention, this can be the perfect time for expanding our minds and our ideas. The growth that takes place now can be incredibly exciting and fulfilling. What a place and what a time to launch this second part of our lives, with the first half now a firm foundation on which to build!

What if we looked forward to retirement only to find that we're not really happy, or filled with a sense of purpose but see all the free time as something to fill rather than to savor? What if we find that the partner we have shared so many of our years with has found someone else – or that we have? What if we realize that we're still carrying around emotional baggage we might have dropped some time ago, but we just don't know how to let go? What if we understand rationally that we don't really need the larger house that served us so well when our family was growing up, but don't know where to move and are not sure we really want to? What if we're

> *"By the time you become fifty, you begin to feel that maybe you might know where you're going."*
>
> – TED EGRI

> *"I upset my security every once in a while. I think it's important that you create a purpose if you don't have one. The one big problem with a society with too much comfort is that you start losing your identity and I think crises are actually necessary for growth."*
>
> – DALE AMBURN

simply afraid of making what appears to be a life change? All of these questions are common ones that are simply outer manifestations of internal dilemmas that arise for many of us. Sometimes these situations that may appear uncomfortable or carry negative connotations may be exactly what we need to get us moving in a different way.

Perhaps awareness and consciousness have already been important components of your life, but never had the chance to expand as they can now. When we do focus on the inner self, we recognize the importance of having that self be a healthy one, one that's not subordinated to the needs of others, but is aware of them in a more balanced way. That is, not to succumb to that which is imposed upon us from the outside, but to honor that part of ourselves that is truly in touch with a more universal truth.

"I realized that expressing my inner feelings and utilizing the most important things in life to fulfill oneself as being one of the most important activities."

One of the ways we can bring that about is to be more of an observer, by taking the time to see what's around us and appreciate the beauty that surrounds us. By taking the time "to smell the roses," watch the changing light in the sky, look at the smile of joy on someone's face, we ourselves are enhanced. It allows us to be more tolerant, perhaps, than we've been before and less critical because we don't necessarily have the same expectations we've previously held. By not imposing them as much upon ourselves, we are less likely to impose them upon others.

"My sculpture really blossomed as a form of protest against inhumanity and injustice."

"I began to see not just the horrors of inhumanity, but I also began to see the beauty. I began to see the Native American people, the Hispanic people and their cultures - the mountains, the depth, the climate - the way things were built around here, so everything became something more positive."

– TED EGRI

Recognizing the finer qualities of people rather than focusing on the negative ones represents another way we can shift our perspective and expand our hearts as well as our minds. Sometimes letting go of so much thinking can be a blessed relief, and as we lower our demands and expectations of others, we can do the same of ourselves. Trying to please everyone (often an accultur-ated feminine trait) no longer may seem quite as important as it is to be true to ourselves. Trusting our intuition more and relying on "information" less may reinforce confidence in our own abilities to make decisions.

"I've slowed down in many of the attitudes that I had. I think I've become more tolerant, more aware of what the good things are all about."

– HELEN ABRAMOWITZ

When we find ourselves more able to shift our perspective, we allow more space for other things to enter our minds and our hearts. Often, we'll find feelings of thankfulness and abundance come flooding in, filling us with a strong sense of well-being. It's very possible that our financial status hasn't improved, but we can feel, at this stage of life, that it really doesn't seem to matter as much as it once did. Not only do we not need all the "stuff" we once may have thought important, but we really don't want it. The appreciation of what we do have will often far outweigh the yearnings we might have had earlier for that which we didn't have. We may discover that many of the things that bring us joy and fulfillment are not material at all, beyond taking care of our basic needs and providing a more "realistic" comfort zone.

"It seemed quite natural that after Bob, my husband, was gone that I would explode, which is what I've done. It's like I've erupted!"

– ANN ST. JOHN HAWLEY

With many of our responsibilities having already been met, a certain time of freedom now presents itself, when we are less caught up in "providing" for others. Now those specific "others" may be providing for themselves and we can take the time that is given to us to step back and see ourselves more for who we are, rather than identify with the roles. When we can let go of those roles and place less emphasis on what we "do" (wife, mother, husband, father, business executive, teacher, longshoreman), we have more of a capacity to see how we "be."

"It took me a little while to realize I didn't have to do anything for anybody – my spiritual life, that's first ... the way I live my life, which is as simple as I can make it."

"Don't you think you need plenty of silence?"

– ANN ST. JOHN HAWLEY

This may also be a time of your life when, if you haven't already become involved, you might become interested in meditation. For so many years our focus has been outward, in "being in the world," so the chance to shift our attention inward may be very welcome. Somehow or other, at this time, we become more introspective, looking at where we are, where we've been, and where we're going. It may represent a time of healthy reevaluation that occurs when the focus turns inward. We might be very grateful for the respite of focusing on the external, and in recognizing more time for ourselves, we might discover that meditation serves as a way of finding that place where we can empty our minds and allow ourselves simply to be.

Meditation means many things to many people. To some it is a formal discipline, developed over many years. But whatever it is that you do, it involves "quieting the mind." The ceaseless chatter that takes place in the mind, the dialogues, the scenarios, the worry and anxiety, the planning and controlling of situations, the concern with the outcome of those plans, are all the favorite activities of the mind. It has not been trained to find a place of quiet, of stillness, of centeredness.

By using a specific technique designed for this purpose of "emptying" the mind, we can lose our attachment to these thoughts and train ourselves to note them as they enter the mind, and then let them go. Surely all of us can remember the many times when it seemed that the ceaseless flow of thoughts took control of us, and we were helpless to stop them. We can almost see ourselves as being hostages of these thoughts spinning out of control, unwilling to have them continue, but finding that often they seemed intent on going their own way.

Techniques for meditation are expressed in various ways, from "sitting" in a particular position for a proscribed period of time, to chanting mantras, to focusing on one's breath. But whatever technique is used, the purpose is the same. Some find themselves comfortable in groups such as in Zen centers, while others have developed their own time and their own format at home, often incorporating yoga, chi gong or other forms of meditation through movement. Like exercise, food and paying attention to your body, paying attention to your mind requires a certain level of consciousness, and it, too, requires commitment in order to be successful.

"The head is not always in touch with the body. You may think you're well and are not, and vice versa ... Eastern religions stress unity of mind, body and spirit."

– DALE AMBURN

For many years I've been somewhat obsessed by dead or dying leaves on plants. There are many plants in the house, and I can usually spot a dead leaf from across the room and, like a beam, I focus on that particular leaf or leaves, and head toward it without any thought. Since I travel several times a year, I know that when I come home, I have to get the plants groomed before I can feel comfortable. But is it really an obsession or simply my own form of meditation? In the summer I can spend hours weeding which I love to do. And when I'm weeding, it's not a question of purposely escaping the thought process. This happens naturally as a by-product of my immersion in what I'm doing. I think of nothing else but the next weed. Sometimes it's hard to say what's compulsive and what becomes a meditation. I think the difference is the sense of focus and the consciousness and awareness engaged.

"The change has taken place from a negative to positive vibration."

– DALE AMBURN

"I'm my own person, but I think this comes with age. It's something you acquire. I became gentler, I don't have anger, which is a destructive thing."

– HELEN ABRAMOWITZ

Just taking time to be focused on the moment, emptying the mind and making space for "nothingness" to enter becomes easier when one acquires the ability that comes through practice, whatever that practice might be. Part of my practice is simply allowing myself that "quiet" space – one of the luxuries of this time of life.

A little about mind-sets. We know that depression, negative emotions, stress, tension and anxiety take a toll emotionally and physically and also deplete us spiritually for they sap our energy, leaving us less vibrant and "alive." Reversing that takes effort, sometimes more than we think we have. But we do have it, we have that power, and through the exercising of that power we can transform something that is negative and destructive into something that is positive and constructive. In so doing, we can become our own alchemists. In orchestrating this transmutation from that which does not serve us to something that is of value can be very self-empowering. How can we enter into a state of harmony and balance if our psychic space is occupied with worry and anxiety? It's not so much what happens to us, it's how we deal with it.

Learn how to set the mind at rest when you need to, rather than have it go off on tangents that use up energy in a non-constructive way such as obsessing on situations that make you feel angry, jealous or anxious. Use the same energy to get to that place of "centeredness." When the mind is in motion, try to maintain a level of consciousness and state of awareness rather than have your thoughts take over and control you. Most of us would so much rather feel good than feel bad, be in a state of happiness, rather than dis-ease. But, like everything else, we have to do our part, we have to want to make the change in our state of mind and help bring that about through purpose and intent. Once that psychic space is provided, you might be very surprised at what can enter.

Plants transform carbon monoxide into oxygen as a normal occurrence. They are designed by nature to perform this function. This is an example of how energy can be changed from one form to another. We, too, can transform negative energy into positive energy. Not only is it an exercise of our own personal power (as opposed to power over another) but it also makes us a copartner with what might be termed "a greater force." If we are to believe there are infinite numbers of possibilities beyond calculation that can occur, I feel it is an obligation to take charge of our own decisions when we're provided with the opportunity to do so.

It's easy to see how our bodies can respond to exercise and healthy diet. What about our thoughts? If, in expanding our consciousness, we train our minds to eliminate negative thoughts as much as possible (unless they provide us with valuable insights and understanding), and focus instead upon those that are constructive, can we not achieve a higher level of mindfulness? As important as it is to keep our muscles strong and our bodies flexible, it is imperative that our minds, too, are kept strong and

"I enjoy experiencing everything,"

– HELEN ABRAMOWITZ

flexible. This happens naturally when we maintain a sense of "openness" to situations, people, life styles, opportunities and changes. By developing and maintaining feelings of compassion, tolerance, caring, loving and sharing, we enrich and expand our selves.

This can be the time of our lives when we can take the opportunity to do some of the things we've always wanted to in a non-judgmental way. We can learn how to sail, build furniture, make stained glass, sing opera or write poetry. Issues such as whether or not we're good at it, whether or not it's frivolous (not of deep meaning), contribute to what we view as necessary, or brings financial remuneration, no longer need to carry the weight they might have during an earlier part of our life. The "I wish I had" can become "Now I can." Seems pretty liberating to me! Growth on every level is part of an ongoing process, or we would find ourselves stagnating. Real personal growth, however, takes place when we meet challenges consciously and find ourselves enriched by them through our ability to learn from and utilize them, and discover within ourselves a deeper level of maturity.

"I like discovering new things."

"We can do anything, we don't have to be tied to one thing."

– Ann St. John Hawley

"If I wanted to recognize age as a factor in my well-being, maybe I would be a couch potato or just a grandma ... I'm certainly not just a cookie grandma. I have a life of my own."

– Helen Abramowitz

Chapter Ten
New Opportunities

*F*or those of us who are grandparents, giving to grand-children of our time and attention and receiving from them their smiles and laughter can be one of the greatest joys we are gifted with. When our own kids were young we were probably so busy trying to make a living and support us all, or take care of our homes and provide for their basic needs, that often the years just slipped away without offering either our children or ourselves the quality of time together that we can now appreciate with our grandchildren. We also seem to be a lot more tolerant of our grandchildren, who are gener-ally with us for comparatively brief periods.

(Last night I dreamed not of my children, but of my grand-children being here at this wonderful place in the Yucatan Peninsula of Mexico to share in what gives me so much plea-sure – the tropical climate, the beauty of the pristine waters of Laguna Bacalar, the sound of the birds, the peace and tran-quility). Taking them to the movies or to a museum, exploring lakes or mountains, taking trips or whatever it is we think would be enjoyable for them as well as us, is a gift of sharing. One of our favorite activities is rock-hunting (a little easier in the mountains than the city – but cities have their own adventures and special places). Not only because it's exciting for us to discover "special" rocks, but because it's a time of being outdoors together, away from TV and computer games. It also shifts their focus from their everyday world, filled with objects of technology to the more natural one.

Now, too, is an ideal time for us to relax not only with what we have, but to begin new projects, take a new path, participate in new activities, discover things that we think we'd enjoy doing, not necessarily those that we feel we "need" to do. That's freedom! And anything we can do to set the soul free allows it to take form and maybe even learn to fly! For when the spirit within us expands, it is the finest form of growth.

Maybe some of that can come about through discovering a new career. Some people have a real fear of losing their jobs and their means of livelihood around this age, having to compete with younger men and women who have more diverse skills, vitality and strength. But often, many men are grateful that their days of sitting behind a desk, swinging a pickaxe, or just working at jobs that have become stale and old or filled with stress and tension, are coming to an end. Rather than worry about how they look and question whether or not they're still "attractive," many women now cherish the security of maturity and happily rediscover the importance of women in their lives, as sisters and friends. All of us can recognize opportunities to make new beginnings. Why not go out and have a new career, make a job change, do something you've never done before, or train for something that interests you, that challenges your mind?

"When I came here (Taos), that was when I decided this was my turn to do what I wanted to do."

— Pat Stallcup

What if you've picked up computer skills that can open up careers that might have been out of reach for you during an earlier part of your life, like designing brochures, writing travel copy, starting a small new business that allows for a more mellow and stress-free life style but still provides the kind of autonomy you like? Reading, writing, and even what used to be called arithmetic can be developed or expanded upon, used in new ways, to provide an alternative to a previous career, profession or job.

The ability to solve problems with greater ease and clarity sometimes makes the role of a consultant one that can be appealing in mid-life, where experience can not only be a valuable asset in freeing oneself from responsibilities of full time work but still contribute the expertise to enable the more relative freedom of consulting work. Some people I know have made important contributions in being involved in fund raising, an activity that might be more feasible now when there may be more free time to devote to this kind of activity. All kinds of volunteer work may be another avenue to explore, with the sense of personal worth and fulfillment being the "rewards."

So many of us are artists, in one area or another, but have never been considered "professionals" since it didn't provide us with the way we made our living. What about just

"I was always an artist."

– Ann St. John Hawley

making art for ourselves as our own individual expression, or discovering projects we might not have thought about before that are artfully designed?

Some people decide that they really love to dance and join groups, or take lessons. To some, it may be the preferred way to exercise. Dance can be extended to some of the oriental disciplines of yoga, tai chi, chi gong, or even karate.

Remember all those doodles you used to make in the margins of your high school notebooks?

Maybe now's the time to invest in some drawing or painting materials and see what happens. Finding a gallery to represent you and get your work out to the public may be ego fulfilling, but won't you be equally as happy in just the "doing" of it? As a matter of fact, what a nice place to be when you can have your ego trade places with your spirit (if you haven't already done so), putting your spirit out front and placing the ego on the "back burner." Chances are, your ego has already had its "up front" time, anyway.

Very often gardening magazines, especially the advertisements in them, feature middle aged folks with trowel in hand. Undoubtedly, for many ages, the appeal of gardening is a major lure, but now we might finally have the time and attention to pay to make gardening another art form. Planting and seeing things grow or producing fruit, vegetables or flowers can only be just a part of it. There are many areas in which we can see our creative ideas become manifested. We can be involved in arranging artistic plantings, building decks or porches, designing ponds or, if we're limited in space, creating specialty gardens, like cactus or bonsai, or even growing orchids in our bathrooms. Does it really matter if our gardens don't end up looking like the ones in the magazines (lots of the ones I find myself entranced by were photographed in some warm, wet climate, and I live in a cold, dry one), as long as we find that the creating part is what excites us, or gives us a feeling of pleasure and satisfaction?

Music has always had a way of speaking to us, which has been evidenced in every culture. Perhaps we might have harbored a secret yearning to be a musician, but for various reasons (like thinking we never really had the talent, or the chances of financial success were too slim to make it a reasonable option in our lives), we never pursued it very seriously. Now with the luxury of middle years, we might take music lessons, learn to play an instrument, or join or form a band. Just the pleasure of doing it for ourselves is really all we need and how wonderful not to have to be concerned with recognition or having our talents judged.

Now can be a time for community involvement and participating in activities taking place in your immediate surroundings, or even going out into the world to lecture and share what you can with others. I know people who've received a great deal of satisfaction becoming involved with people in prison, with Habitat for Humanity, and even joining the Peace Corps. By now, we probably have a pretty good notion of what's needed to help others, and many of us now have the time to recognize that

"I've always, since my college years, been interested in service – humans are the only animals who can choose to serve."

– BILL STALLCUP

desire and do something about it. With the benefit and knowledge acquired from so many of life's experiences, we can truly start sharing that with others, from helping raise money for what we consider worthy causes, to providing moral support to those willing and able to receive it. Sometimes discovering new interests of our own places us in that position of being able to share them with others who might have similar interests. It might even provide them with the necessary motivation for doing something they didn't know how to make happen on their own and provide the needed inspiration.

Travel has held a lot of attraction for people of all ages, but it's something else we might have put off for a variety of reasons, or if we have had travel experiences, we may have yearned for the opportunity to do some more of it. Now we might have the time and financial resources to do that. One part of the travel scenario is that it might encourage us to learn a new language, which is no doubt more of a challenge at this time of our lives than when we were in school. But for what we might be lacking on a neuro-physiological level (that is, in the diminishing of the secretion of the fluids that conduct messages in that part of the brain which is involved in language), we probably make up for in enthusiasm and willingness to learn. And even if we don't ever speak the other language with the fluency we're used to in our own, as long as we can make ourselves understood, haven't we accomplished something? After living part of each year for the past thirty years in Mexico, I still don't speak grammatically correct Spanish, but somehow I don't let that stop me from experiencing a good part of my life in that country. That means not only enjoying the climate and scenery, which may be different, but connecting with people in authentic ways, through sharing our feelings, relating our stories.

At one time travel was restricted to a particular class of person who had both the money and the time, or to the adventurer who made the time and didn't care about the money, or to those who were in military or company service and sent somewhere other than their own country at someone else's behest. Now travel, like communication, has become much more available to a greatly expanded populace. If you've gotten to the point that you can qualify, chronologically speaking, to be a "senior citizen." you get all kinds of benefits. Personally, I feel this is only just, as there has to be something else to reaching this age than more lines in the face or graying hair! Yes, we should be encouraged to travel, and the monetary incentives like substantially reduced air fares or discounts in hotels and motels can make those travel dreams become a reality. Travel doesn't necessarily mean staying at first class hotels in major capitols around the world. It can mean exploring places that used to be considered remote, trekking or archeological exploration of preceding cultures we know little about. It can be travel with a companion, with a group, or alone.

Meeting other people in other countries can be a revelation and a rich source of personal experience of other perspectives, food, climate and landscapes. Also travel within one's own country can be a new experience and an exciting one. The benefit there is you already speak the language, and for some the sense of security of knowing that you're in your own country, within easy access of friends or relatives, can be an important one. Whatever it is that you choose to do, wherever it is that you go, it could become an important part of your life, expanding your vistas at a time when you might be better able to take advantage of the opportunities.

Lots of people now are so mobile that often families are located in many different regions or perhaps different countries and visits with them can provide an exciting and enriching form of "travel." There can not only be time spent with our friends and relations but these trips can provide a nice reason for an extended stay in an area we might have known nothing about, incorporating a visit with exploration. I've always loved flowers and trees and bushes and anything that's green and growing, but except for one visit to Buschart Gardens on Vancouver Island in British Columbia, I've not really seen any "formal" botanical gardens. Recently we talked with a friend, who has similar feelings for gardens, about just taking a two or three day trip to a well known botanical garden in our region, staying at a nice B&B, and making it a mini-vacation. Some times just a theme or special interest is enough to help you plan an itinerary, whether it's visiting gardens, spas or birth-sites of famous poets.

What's really there for us now is an opportunity to break old patterns that are no longer fulfilling or satisfying, replacing them instead

"Some of the people we know, they continue, even after they're retired, in the same patterns doing the same things because that's the only thing they know, and they seem to be lost without those attachments and activities – they can't let go. If you're only involved in social activities, in that which "others" do, it doesn't work, because then you don't have a life of your own."

– PAT STALLCUP

"I call myself an old lady, but I don't feel old!"

– ANN ST. JOHN HAWLEY

with those that are positive and enriching and are a means to further personal growth. If something doesn't work for us any more, we have other choices, alternatives to be explored. In spite of the fact that we live in a youth oriented society with such an emphasis on consumerism, there are some wonderful benefits to these next fifty years. One of them is that we generally are more self-confident and no longer suffer from a need to achieve certain goals, conform to particular patterns of accepted life styles, and in general focusing on the need to build for the future. Perhaps that might mean greater focus on where we are now in this present moment.

Chapter Eleven
Reading, Writing
(No Arithmetic)

*F*or those for whom reading is one of life's great pleasure, isn't this a superb opportunity to take the time to read old classics, or new books by some of the marvelous contemporary authors producing works that introduce us to other perspectives and insights or stories that touch us in a meaningful way? These might have just passed us by back in the days when it seemed our lives were so taken up by other things we deemed to be more important. There just wasn't the time for that kind of luxury! But reading can be a rich and satisfying experience now and can cover an extensive array of material.

Reading for pleasure is a wonderful indulgence. We find ourselves transported and hear the voice of the author speaking to us through the characters depicted or the stories that are being told, becoming immersed in what has been created for us through the written word. Like self-help books that have found

"Everybody speaks with poetry. The whole thing is that you have to find the way to do it. What I want to do is let go, not remain in a stationary position. This represents my sense of freedom."

– Ann St. John Hawley

such a receptive audience, there seems to be more room for the publishing of fine new novels, poems and short stories, as well as translations from previously obscure mystic writers like Rumi and John of the Cross. We now have access, as we've never had before, to new writers as well as established writers who have an expanded market to appreciate their work. And what a complete luxury it can be to be able to read at night and not fall asleep after the first couple of pages because you're exhausted having spent the majority of your day taking care of your kids, your home, your job. With fewer demands made upon our time, we can afford the feeling of "indulging" ourselves in more extensive reading. And, for the devoted reader, is there not a wonderful feeling of "wealth" when we have several books piled up on our nightstand, just waiting to be enjoyed!

"I'm pretty much a studier – I like to work, investigate things, read things that are going on, teach myself."

– Pat Stallcup

Many of us who are readers are writers as well. Sometimes we're aware of it, sometimes we're not. Some who might never have jotted down a thought, written a poem or experimented with a screen play, may now find themselves captivated by this means of self-expression. The wonderful part of getting this kind of "late start," is that it's not necessarily tied to ideas of a career or personal recognition, but more for self-satisfaction. You don't even have to care whether or not it's "good," for judgment by critics may have nothing to do with this endeavor. Sometimes joining a writing group can provide both the stimulus and the support you find to be just what you need to get going. Like a spa, gym or health club, we might initially back off from group participation, feeling we might not have the necessary talent or ability or that others have had more experience or might be better at it. So what? People who share a philosophical approach to being in groups are probably not competitive, but are ready, willing and able to have someone of like mind participate in the sharing of what you and others have to offer.

Some of us have been writing for a long time but have found that the ordinary activities of life seemed always to take precedence over writing. Yet we've felt the creative urge often, and may have reams of written material to prove it. These years can provide just that opportunity we've been waiting for to seriously apply ourselves to that form of self-expression. Just as Grandma Moses didn't start painting until she was in advanced years, many people in their mid-years discover that they have something to say and can say it well through poetry, novels, memoirs, journals of personal experiences or specific areas of interest like birding or archeology, flower arranging or building fountains.

> *"I'm one of those people who have to climb the mountain, whether anyone else cares or not. I'm one of those people who writes poetry whether anyone else ever reads it or not."*
>
> – DALE AMBURN

What makes a writer is like asking what makes a painter or musician. Is it the talent inherent within us, or simply the participation in the expression of the art form? Is it based on years of experience developing our craft, finding new techniques, or is it the willingness to experiment with the unknown and finding out what happens? Is it the reviews we read in the papers that motivate us, or is it simply "doing it!" as writer Natalie Goldberg says, that brings us all the reward we need?

The gap between generations can be more extensive than we realize. Our generation, in particular, has seen major changes, primarily in the field of electronics, communication and transportation. With the enormous growth of population, villages, towns and cities have gone through tremendous transitions with great import sociologically and economically. The opportunities and choices offered have made relocation a way of life, impacting significantly upon family structure, so that the previous support systems and caregiving by relatives has often become a thing of the past and coming up with new ways to deal with these changes can be challenging. Now, not every family has the luxury of close daily contact with the different generations. But when they do, it can be a nice time of exchange, especially between grandparents and their grandchildren.

"I try to be with young people because they're inspiring and because I enjoy them. I refuse to become old, in the sense of old meaning I have to depend on others, complaining, thinking only of myself. I don't want that, there's too much ahead, there's too much to learn. I'm writing now, my memoirs, a treasury of memories."

– HELEN ABRAMOWITZ

One of the things that children everywhere love to hear about is how times were when their parents were children, because until they get to an age of reason it's almost impossible to relate to the fact that their parents and grandparents were once children too. Writing about your own experiences when you were a child can be a source of pleasure to your grandchildren who have never known a world without air travel, computers and television. Telling stories orally is a form of writing, too, which might come under the heading of reminiscences to you, but paints a picture through words for them.

I suppose I've wanted to write ever since I can remember. It seems that I always had a pen or pencil in hand, with which to write or draw. Writing became a little easier when I got into high school for that's what you were supposed to do, at least in English class. That of course was my favorite subject and the only one I was really interested in. By the time I was a senior I had received some criticisms on poetry I had written, including "this is good, is it yours?" That comment not only felt scathing but unjustified and more than a little annoying.

However this same teacher was one of the ones who judged our anonymous senior essays. Mine was largely written in a soda shop, where as a special escape from peanut butter sandwiches I would indulge, with my friends, in a weekly extravaganza of a hamburger, french fries and a cherry coke. Although like most of us who somewhere in their hearts holds the hope that they will be acknowledged, both my friends and I were somewhat astounded when my name actually was called at a school assembly to receive an award for the senior essay contest. I experienced the thrill of recognition for an ability to express, through the written word, that which I had done for my own pleasure or need for self-expression. It was the affirmation that other people could possibly hear what I had to say, for it was so much easier to write these thoughts than to speak them.

Fifteen years and a family later, these thoughts remained with me and became more amplified with my life experiences as an adult, mother, wife, and citizen of the world. My sense of "connectedness" that was the focus of my high school essay was stronger than ever and my sense of dissatisfaction with the way people treated each other, the prevailing political climate and the rampant consumerism that had already become apparent reflected values that seemed shallow, lacking in authenticity. The death of my eldest son when he was ten and a half years old seemed to reinforce in my personal life that which I saw in the outside world, events that didn't make sense. But it also provided the impetus to pursue something I had never finished. So I went back to school.

Because I didn't have all the necessary requirements due to some "holes" in my high school education, I had to take a few qualifying courses, but the college credits I received by taking some exams, based on my own personal knowledge in specific subjects, made up for some of the credits I was lacking. When I completed my two years at a community college with an associate degree transferable to a university, I felt that I could now set about doing what I really wanted to, which was to design my own program based on my particular needs with a specific project in mind.

That was the start of my understanding that I could, in certain arenas, take charge of how I could make things happen in spite of the obstacles that were presented to me and, at the same time, create the opportunity of expressing my own insights based on life experience and reflective thought. After experimenting with several areas of study, I found them all to be lacking in the "holistic" view I held until I came to philosophy. Finally, there was a course of study that felt it encompassed just about everything. But rather than immerse myself in the study of different philosophers and their specific systems, I found that particular ways of thought felt compatible to my intuitive understanding and, like a hummingbird, I went from flower to flower gleaning my own nourishment. I discovered the work of the German existential phenomenologist, Martin Heidegger, and became introduced to Buddhist thought, both of which resonated with what I felt to be my truth.

Looking for alternatives to the lifestyle that was familiar to me, I was fortunate to find a visiting professor emeritus to sponsor me and designed a program based on two years of interviews with people who had chosen lifestyles other than those of the prevailing ones. Most of these alternative situations were still experimental and many were changing and adapting to the new problems they encountered. So, in addition to taking one or two courses each semester on campus, I traveled to various parts of the region being with various groups of people until I, along with my husband, decided to make a major change in our own lives. But now writing had once more entered my life and after I had completed my studies, I set off with my family to a remote area in Mexico with the express purpose of writing about what I had observed in researching this "project."

While I was busy making plans, life happened. Like everyone, I underwent many life changes and writing got placed on the back burner, with a new relationship on the front burner. With a new part of my life unfolding, recording didn't seem nearly as important as the experiencing. Writing didn't really happen again until another long hiatus of many years. Then, somewhere, somehow, poetry started to emerge, usually randomly, when the "urge" possessed me. After the abrupt (they never really are) break-up of a twenty-two year relationship, I found myself journaling. It wasn't anything I had to think about. It was my natural tool to express my thoughts and feelings, the imperative of the spirit, long suppressed. I was sixty-two.

So there we have it! Writing, as all art forms, must be recognized as the spirit's way of claiming acknowledgement. Flashes of that had occurred all through my life, but outside "distractions" managed to take dominance over that form of expression. This beautiful spirit that dwelled within seemed to be perfectly happy, never attempting to force its way onto my conscious life, just patiently abiding. We each have this internal spirit that seems to demand that its presence be known, sometimes urgently, or perhaps quietly and subtly. It provided those flashes of clarity, of manifesting that kind of knowing we refer to as intuition. Often this is not so much in the form of "saying" something, but simply through the expression of a feeling, an emotion or insight that comes from a place other than the conscious mind.

Writing means different things to different people. It seems that all of my life I've been taking notes in my mind, observing and recording. We each have our own stories, our own feelings, observations and experiences. They constitute the fabric that makes up our lives. Writing is not necessarily for others to read, although if they felt they wanted to share it, it would be like a new friendship. It really presents itself to us from that place of spirit based on intuition, manifesting as creativity, that says, "I'm here."

Chapter Twelve
Sex & Consumerism

*T*he term "mid-life crisis" has lots of connotations. Although it frequently seems to revolve around sexual issues, that appears to be just part of an overall re-evaluation that often takes place at this time. It's not surprising that this sexual aspect becomes a primary focus. With all the beautiful young women depicted on magazine covers having "fun" (which is always what they're doing in commercials), there is both an obvious and subliminal suggestion that the way to express your need for freedom may be with a distinct focus on the sexual aspect. If you're male, it appears that you too could have this kind of life (sexy looking women). If you're female and look like they do, the suggestion is that you, too, would be having "fun." Some people, although mature in many ways, seem to buy the symbol still – fast sports cars, a different style of dressing, acting "cool." But if acting is involved, it can't be very authentic (unless you're getting paid to perform professionally, as in the theater or movie industry). However, if it's not authentic it won't hold up in the long run.

The emphasis on sexuality is rampant in our society. Cartoon characters on children's television programs that depict the powerful "wonder-woman" image (or even evil spirit incarnate) with tiny waistlines and oversized breasts can establish, at a very early age, what is deemed "desirable" in a woman, setting the stage for a mind set that is constantly reinforced by continued advertising assaults. How many billboards have we seen advertising a variety of products that feature attractive young women with accentuated cleavage in larger-than-life images that have nothing whatsoever to do with the products being sold?

At one time magazine covers would depict a variety of backgrounds and subject matters that related to what would be found inside. Now, virtually every magazine, whether it's about auto mechanics or fashion, uses that image of the well endowed, overly exposed, beautiful young woman, giving support to the notion "it sells!" Even articles that are written about a broad spectrum of subjects often use the same kind of attention getting device. We often see attractive young men included (but rarely featured), telling us that as females we can probably attract that kind of guy if we just wore the right kind of jeans. Or as males we can probably attract that superb feminine image if we drove the right kind of car. But, basically, that's what they are – images. The only emphasis they provide is on the physical aspect of what our culture has deemed desirable.

One would think that our society is the first one to discover sexuality. Maybe it's the first one to use it and exploit it to the extent we see today for our society is based on consuming products and if sex helps sell them, it is the method of choice. What's really interesting is that we rank among the top in western societies for teenage pregnancies and the preponderance of single mothers is overwhelming. We often bemoan these statistics but fail to see the connection between the statistics and the excessive promotional assault, using sexual stimuli, in our everyday lives.

How does this impact upon our later years? Often we find people past fifty falling into a couple of different categories: those who like to think of themselves as young and "attractive" (meaning sexually), or those who feel those days are over for them and make no effort to retain their vitality (not necessarily sexual). Somehow or other, recognized consciously or not, sex becomes an issue to deal with. Neither one of these attitudes may have the kind of validity we think of as authentic, but they become an area or issue on which to focus, a leftover from earlier stages of our personal identification when many young people base their feelings of personal worth on their ability to attract the opposite sex.

The market for those who would like to think of themselves as young and attractive in this way is enormous. All kinds of creams and treatments abound, suggesting that if we only used the referred to products we, too, will look like the models in these ads (if we're female). How they can get women past fifty and sixty to identify with women who are in their twenties is as amazing as the old ploy used by itinerant hustlers selling snake oil to "cure" all kinds of ailments. Exercise programs, which really are a sound part of keeping physically fit, often appeal to both men and women as a way of keeping their bodies more attractive specifically to maintain their sexual attractiveness. And even the folks bringing us all kind of diet supplements (including natural ones) really can go to town using young, sexy models as an impetus to be more appealing sexually, rather than emphasizing the health benefits to shedding excess weight.

For those who fall into this category of wanting to retain their sexual attractiveness, we also have a fertile field for surgcal implants in areas felt to be lacking, reductions in areas we deem excessive, and attenuating cosmetic procedures of all kinds to remake us into the image that has been promoted virtually all our lives. The market seems to be primarily aimed at women, but it really appeals to both sexes, women because they have been convinced they need conform to the sexual image that has been promoted and men, as well, for buying into that image. Thus, it becomes self-perpetuating.

For thousands of years of recorded history, in every society, older men have been depicted with younger women, whether in harems or with third or fourth wives (this last approach doesn't get rid of the first wife, but simply supplements her). It's certainly more rare that older women are involved with younger men. So, is it any wonder that women today feel they have to do whatever it takes to maintain their position, vying with women who may be twenty or thirty years younger than they are? The whole situation relies on insecurity and power – those who feel, because of a lack of inner security, that their ability to be sexually attractive is what really counts and those who feel, because of the same lack of inner security, that the ability to attract someone "hot" is a proof of their (sexual) power. What a market!

Now we get to those who have neither the inclination nor motivation to deal with the problem of aging and losing their "sexuality." They, too, identify with sexual attraction as being something of acknowledged importance, but they lament their situation rather than deal with it. They still haven't gotten it – that being attractive sexually is not necessarily based on how they look, but rather on their overall vitality, self esteem and internal spirit. They accept it as part of what happens when "you're over the hill," not seeing the beautiful valley on the other side of that hill.

Some of the most vital, attractive people I know are in their fifties and sixties. They take care of themselves on a physical level, but their vitality is an expression of their mental states, their creativity and their spiritual connection to the innermost part of their being. I've never discussed with them their sex lives, but none of them seem to focus on that aspect.

Perhaps they have a satisfying sex life with a partner, or perhaps they are quite happy either abstaining or with a good deal of modification in the kind of sexual activity that was part of a different stage of their lives.

One of the things that occurs as we get older is that endorphins start to replace the previously high hormone levels of estrogen and testosterone. Those hormones are designed with the express purpose of stimulating the act of procreation. As we age (way before we reach our fifties), the production of these hormones slows down and by the time we are in our middle years, we find instead that the endorphins are kicking in. Now that we don't have to be concerned about reproducing, we might feel satisfied with cuddling and nearness providing feelings of warmth and contentment. For those who have spouses or partners, just lying in bed holding each other may be all the sex they need.

The issue of impotence can be something for mature, caring partners to look at from a different perspective. It obviously affects both men and women, for somehow many people feel that their need to "perform" sexually reflects their ability to express love in certain proscribed ways, valid at an earlier time of their lives. It can also reflect a feeling of insecurity if looked at from an "ego" point of view, when all that might be needed is a place of loving understanding and acceptance.

For those who live alone, the warmth of being with good friends, sharing a meal, curling up with a good book, often satisfies the needs that previously would have focused on a romantic encounter. Romance, too, may be undergoing a shift in our understanding. As a species, we tend to romanticize many things, from sexual attraction to success in the market place, to producing a great artistic work. We can see this notion still at play in advertising but at this point in our lives, our notions of romance and sexuality may be far different than they once were.

Our values in general are probably due for an overhaul, which is why we frequently find ourselves questioning on a deeper level what is really important at this time. Often values that we've developed and held on to over the years no longer seem valid, while some still endure. It's a good time to eliminate what no longer applies, to rethink consumerism and to establish our own values about what's really of importance. If your primary concerns becomes overall health and well-being, keeping your body, mind and spirit balanced and in harmony and taking the time and energy to be as fully present in all that you do, you may create a shift in your value system that can impact upon the rest of your life.

If we rethink "consumerism," what it takes and has taken to provide all the material things we might have or wanted to acquire, and apply that same energy towards living a healthier and happier life in general, we've already reduced lots of pressures and tensions. If we can strive to succeed at being the best we are rather than acquiring prestige or success that is measured only by monetary rewards, we may find happiness and tranquility to be much more valuable than a new car or expensive clothes. That, too, may represent an important shift in values. In the kind of consumer society that is prevalent now, we're bombarded from the earliest age with advertisements specifically aimed at maintaining constant pressures to buy, whatever it is, from sugared cereals and soft drinks to toys that are programmed to self-destruct. And that's only the beginning, for the small child of today is the adult of tomorrow. Sugared cereals may change to alcohol and the toys may be faster cars, boats, or motorcycles, the bigger and more numerous, the better.

Although much of the advertising is aimed at a young market with models that younger people can more easily identify with, people of these middle years can be a great deal more discriminating. We would like to think that we are more sure of who we are than we might have been when we were in our twenties and thirties. This can represent an important shift in focus. What traits we might previously have deemed to be attractive because of the passions aroused might change to a softer feeling based on comfort, harmony and lack of stress, tension or high drama. What we find appealing now might not reflect so much the "packaging" but recognition and appreciation of internal qualities. In developing more respect for ourselves, we are less likely to conform to ideals and images, but more likely to be attracted to the "real thing."

Section Four
Freeing the Spirit

We raise our individual voices

And the Universe

Responds in harmony

Chapter Thirteen
Inspirational Teachings

*E*ach of the people who have appeared as part of this book is extraordinary in their own way. They exemplify positive attitudes, heightened awareness, honesty and integrity in the way they live their lives. In some ways they are probably not much different from many people you've come across in your own lives, just the individual stories differ. Having people in our lives who inspire us, who through example, guide us in our thinking, showing us how we can deal with our own issues, is a blessing that needs to be recognized and honored. They are the elders who illuminate the paths we too shall travel. If given a choice, we would travel that path with grace, with consciousness, with a sound mind, body and spirit.

When Alvin Toffler wrote his book "Future Shock," in the Fifties, he pointed out the astounding changes that had taken place in the first half of the twentieth century. The acceleration has continued as we find ourselves with another half a century behind us, bringing us theories and practices only just dreamed of earlier, and beyond the imagination of most. Quantum theory has launched new ways of thinking and understanding, and we are only on the frontier of discovering the practical applications. If we think the twentieth century has revolutionized our way of life in one great quantum leap, are we not also involved, whether we are aware of it or not, in a quantum leap of consciousness?

Times of upheaval are always signified as times of transition, for out of the chaos comes change. Something new is created. But many people who feel chaos in their lives may also feel an inability to keep up with all they feel has to be attended to. They may find themselves wondering, "What's it all about?" The competitive need to get ahead, to strive to accumulate things, prestige, comfort, power, recognition, may become tempered as we get older – our perspective often shifts. Some of us know this intuitively and respond by seeking new visions of what it means to satisfy our internal needs. Others respond by trying to hold on to old values, to specific things, lifestyles or the way they look.

If we're lucky enough to have developed the ability to see, we will recognize our teachers. They may be like the people I've described. We may find them in something we read that triggers an important insight. They may be part of an invisible support system ("The Soul's Code" by James Hillman). But what easier way has been given to us than that of our senses, to observe and appreciate the natural mundane world. Here, every moment, we are witness both to the constant state of flux in which we exist and that which remains constant. It is the understanding that although nothing ever stays the same, there is also continuity. Both aspects reflect the essential qualities that describe "that which is."

But we also have another sense, what is sometimes referred to as the sixth sense, real enough that giving it a name gives credence to it's existence. It is through this sense that we intuit on a level no one has ever been able to successfully describe, but has been experienced in every culture, during every time. In the Sixties and Seventies we called this "tuned in." Tuned in to what? Perhaps, it refers to receiving new understandings through insights (and for a lucky few, through revelation or direct transmission), through the perception of life as a metaphor. If we can shape these questions, and then lay them aside, without searching for answers that we probably are not equipped to understand anyway, maybe we can keep ourselves open to receive whatever these teachings have to offer. We certainly know by now that many things we have learned have come to us not in the form of written information or data but by insightful thinking.

Teachers abound. Sometimes we find them in nature. Writers like Henry David Thoreau and Annie Dillard describe their relationship with the natural world with both beauty and wisdom. These kinds of writings have impacted upon many others for generations. We sometimes find these same kinds of insights and ideas that spark our thinking through writers of philosophy, social consciousness, ethics, mysticism or poetry. But that's only one kind of teaching. We often find our insights triggered by others, through acts of caring and compassion. We can discover our teachers in the myriad aspects of our lives. Some of our greatest teachers are our own experiences, frequently the ones we find the most painful, many not of our own choosing. Sometimes we have to ask for teachers to appear and then have the ability to recognize them! Often the recognition doesn't take place until a later time.

Some years ago I found myself alone at a place of spectacular natural beauty called Agua Azul, outside of Palenque in the southern part of Mexico, in Lacandon country. It was during a trip made with the specific purpose of confronting people and places that had been meaningful in my life so that I could come to terms with what I viewed as an ending before I could make a new beginning. Although I was well aware of not having any expectations as far as experiencing a mystical experience through encountering a special guru or guide, I certainly was open to the opportunity of finding that happen.

The day I was at Agua Azul was very different from the day I had been there more than twenty-five years earlier when there was virtually no one there but our family. This day many people were walking alongside the spectacular waterfalls that cascaded down the hill. As I made my way down the rocky dirt path, walking through brambles and exposed roots, I found myself walking behind an elderly Indian man dressed in traditional simple white cotton shirt and pants and sandals. He said nothing but I had the distinct feeling that I was walking in the shadow of a shaman. That was enough. I nodded as I passed him and that was the entire exchange. But I felt good afterward in a quiet way that spoke to that place of stillness of the soul.

We each have not only our specific lessons but have discovered our own universal understandings through our particular experiences and ways of seeing. I recently found a great insight when I was picking dead leaves off the plants. I found myself returning after I thought I had gotten them all, and discovered more each time I looked. I don't believe they appeared suddenly or magically. It simply required a shift in perspective to see them. It's something we all know, often easier to say than to do, and sometimes it takes something like dead geranium leaves to illuminate the principle. Often, this feeling of insight is accompanied by a great "ah-ha!" Something resonates and says, "so that's what it's all about!" Well, perhaps that's not all of what it's about, but maybe it's something of it, an aspect.

One beautiful day in January in northern Arizona, I went hiking with a friend around a crystalline lake high in the mountains. We sat down on the large, flat rocks that lay around the perimeter and found ourselves not only deep in conversation, but also with that quiet space that allows us to look with "different" eyes. The sun was shining on the incredible rock formations that provided the background for the lake, with shadow and light illuminating what appeared to be a special show for us. It was awesome in its beauty. We watched, transfixed, happy in our being together to witness that beauty. Taking a break to comment on what we were seeing, we noticed that when we focused once again on the scene in front of us, the light had changed, and now the foreground was illuminated. As magnificent as the background had been earlier, now the foreground held the same magic. Because our focus was now on what was up close, we were able to see all the incredible details that we were unable to see when our gaze was distanced across the lake.

There was no doubt of the beauty unfolding in front of our eyes, nor was there any doubt of the metaphor being presented to us. Changes in light, shifts in perspective take place all the time. Sometimes, like that day, they're more dramatic, more noticeable. Often they take place on a far more subtle level. What was so much a part of our awareness was the unchanging beauty of the lake. The changing aspect of the light, our attention focused on the foreground or background and the shift of our own perspective and how it affected what we saw as observers were a stunning example of how we view phenomena. It illuminated my understanding of one of the principles of quantum mechanics described by Gary Zukov and others, something I never would have been able to relate to without those readings.

When we participate in the kind of experiences that teach us through affirmation of something we might have read or heard, it allows us to connect with that teaching. It no longer is an abstract idea or image, but something that we can attest to through our own understanding, something we bear witness to and incorporate into our "truth." As human beings with the unique ability to use more than just instinct, but reason and insight, we are constantly given opportunities to apply inspired teachings to that which we experience in our everyday lives. Perhaps one of the reasons we can identify with great teachers and spiritual guides is that they have been more dedicated to getting to that place of illumination, and in so doing, are able to transmit the knowledge of what they have found to others. Sometimes their words are enough to strike a responsive chord, but often it is through our own application of that which has been presented to us and our ability to see through an expanded consciousness, that we can transcend "that which appears to be."

Chapter Fourteen
Collaboration with the Universe

*W*e don't have to be physi-
cists to participate in
understanding Universe. We simply
have to be in partnership with it.
Rather than feel that we are either
completely at the hands of "fate"
or that we are in total control of
our own lives, we've all experienced enough of the process of
living that it becomes apparent
that it's some of both and probably a little bit of something more
we are not yet equipped to understand. This mutual participation
becomes a collaboration where
we do our part, knowing that
other events are taking place
which, luckily or unluckily, really are beyond our control.

This sense of collaboration
becomes the connective conduit.

*"I became more and more
aware of the relationship
between myself and the
universe – I began studying
for myself to see what the
relationship of the human
species has to do with
universal law – scientists
were looking for knowledge
of what is going on in the
universe – if we look into
the human brain, we will
see all the laws of the
universe are to be found
there. All the principals
that exist in the universe
are within all living things.
I, myself, am every living
thing in the universe."*

– TED EGRI

We expend energy and we receive energy, for we are energy in a particular form, which is ever changing, while the consciousness of that which is "I" remains constant. Our bodies change, our personalities change, our values change. As we mature we can see our lives as a tapestry still on the loom, but with enough of the work done to be able to see part of the pattern. We understand the mechanics of how the loom must be threaded first with the warp as the underlying structure. This is the "I-ness." Only then can come the woof, line by line, creating whatever pattern that emerges. Emotions provide the different colors while strength is determined by the tightness of the weave. Sometimes the warp breaks and is tied once again. The weaving can be smooth or it can be textured. Although some patterns resemble others and have elements in common, each is unique. That uniqueness is simply a manifestation of all that takes place in the universe. No combination of neutrons, protons, or electrons can ever be the same. Even when we try to monitor them, that itself impacts upon the configuration and how each component behaves.

None of us can predict what the next fifty years, or balance thereof, will reveal, any more than we could have foreseen for the first fifty. But as we were nourished and guided, perhaps we can be a source of nourishment and guidance. First, however, we must maintain, to the best of our ability, a sense of our own centeredness. This becomes easier to maintain as our natural state of being when our awareness is kept carefully honed, our consciousness not buried under piles of useless debris, but with an open mind that thrives on clarity.

Inherent in the idea of manifesting those things we've always

"I think it's the awareness, it's just to be aware of growing, to be more aware of the fact that we're just a little piece of God. We need to be one with the body which is God. Whatever it is, we need to be part of it, in union with and not feel isolated."

– ANN ST. JOHN HAWLEY

wanted, and creating new ideas and directions, is the concept of "unfoldingness." In past years, we've been so busy living in the world with all the attendant responsibilities that we've often had the tendency to "take charge" of our destinies. We've, quite naturally, been involved in pursuing particular goals such as families, careers, professions and focusing our attention and energies on these directions. We've very often, out of necessity, put our own personal needs on "hold." Sometimes simply keeping our heads above water seemed to take all we had, and more. Stepping back and allowing the time/space for things to unfold didn't always seem possible.

Yet this "unfoldingness" is taking place all the time. The Universe constantly does provide, but what is required between this and the receiving is individual participation. That's the great collaboration that takes place between us and the Universe. To rely solely on one aspect throws things out of balance, and it is difficult to maintain the proper perspective. Now however, at this time of our lives, the second half, we have more opportunity to step back from our attitude of constant directing, and allow this "unfoldingness" to take place. As soon as we make space for the unknown to enter, something surely does.

If we think of ourselves as being an individual cell in a larger organism, as part of the vast, unknown Universe, we need to keep ourselves healthy on every level. Healthy is also happy. A sound mind, body and spirit provides a happy place for the internal spirit to dwell. As we manifest our own energy in the most positive way, so too do we influence the whole. A fit body and an active mind are not enough. Our spirits, too, must be free to become more fully real-

"There's someplace I need to go and I'm going. If you reach the end, you're dead!"

"The spiritual, that's the thing, the spiritual life. Everything we do is spiritual. We are spirit – we're living it."

– Ann St. John Hawley

ized. For this, they need space – if we provide it, that spirit will grow and become strong, taking its place in its connection to the Whole.

Chapter Fifteen
The Moment

*I*t's been hundreds of thousands of years of human evolution since Neanderthal "man," If the human species has evolved to the point we find ourselves at now, what does that say about our concept of time? Obviously, we have very little notion of what the term means, or even if it exists. While we note that great change has taken place, with continual acceleration, over what we consider a vast time span, what changes have been taking place on other levels simultaneously? We are at an exciting time of our individual lives, and perhaps at an exciting time on a much larger scale. As we develop more of a perspective of time and space, with greater understanding becoming available, perhaps it's because only now are we at the point where we're able to receive it. We simply weren't ready a hun-

"Some of the most creative periods in history happen to be periods of turmoil."
– TED EGRI

"I also like chaos. You have to have some chaos in order to find a new way. Although it's painful and you feel lost, out of chaos comes some kind of direction or insights – something new emerges."
– ANN ST. JOHN HAWLEY

dred thousand years ago, or even a thousand years ago. Maybe we just needed the preparation.

It seems to be apparent that great acts of creativity are often triggered by vast upheaval and times of dissention. This is one of the ways we can see change take place. However, things are always operating on subtler levels as well. While some people seem to be peculiarly equipped to act as catalysts, instigating change through the force of their own energy, others seem better equipped to show us the meaning of harmony and balance. Their work may be less dramatic, but they represent the opposite principle of energy in motion. Theirs is energy at rest. When we look at these two principles we see the need for both. As we can recognize our own male and female aspects, so too can we see other dualities, that of participating in change and shifts and that which identifies with what is enduring. We see that we need both to achieve that place of harmony and balance. How static it would be to sit in the middle of a seesaw with no movement. But what would it be like to be in constant motion, extremes of down on the ground, or soaring up in the air, without sometimes coming to that place in the middle?

"One has to become aware of so many things about one that you have no time to think of anything else, just being aware."

"By using many disciplines you get closer to the truth of the world around you which will fulfill our needs, our own personal truth."

– Ted Egri

The more disciplined we are and the more experience we have, the easier it is to return to that point of harmony and balance. By discipline, I don't mean deprivation. When we refuse to take chemically altered foods into our bodies, even if they appear to taste good and our minds might think we'd like to have them, that's not deprivation, it's common sense exercised as discipline. When we get in a consistent amount of conscious exercise that too is not deprivation, but discipline. When we take the time to participate in meditation practices, that does not require deprivation, but discipline. The carpenter who uses his tools with ease and knowledge of what's required, the painter who uses her palette knife or brush without having to think of the next move, have years of discipline behind them. When the technique has been mastered, there is a certain freedom of expression that becomes possible, an ability to go beyond.

One of the great freedoms that become apparent is our understanding of living in the moment. This does not necessarily imply that we have no plans or responsibilities. But it seems that as we reach these middle years with the frequent questioning that accompanies this time of transition, we can see that the expectations of what we think life should be like is often surprisingly different from what actually takes place. If we were able to lessen our attachment to those preconceived notions, it seems we would do ourselves a far better service. When we are more able to savor the individual moments we can see things with a different perspective and the experience of the lessons shown become more apparent. Rather than depend on the seven o'clock news to provide us with information of what's going on in the world, we can make our own determinations based on our own inquiries. Rather than depend on outside entertainment in whatever form it takes to divert our attention, we might find ourselves more focused on going inward to find the satisfaction we seek. We might discover the importance and value of good conversation. That means exchange of ideas, thoughts and feelings in a deep and meaningful way. And rather than think we have answers, we may welcome the opportunity to go beyond the known.

"That's about all I can do as a human being is to glimpse something for a moment, an atom of enrichment."

– ANN ST. JOHN HAWLEY

I love being the age I am now! So what if there are lines in my face; they tell my stories. I love not being caught up in what needs to be done as much as what can be done. When I look at old people, I'm struck by a strong sense of compassion. I know they would deem it a gift to be where I am now, feeling energetic and healthy, my steps strong where theirs falter, my health vigorous where theirs may have become fragile. Let us celebrate this time of our lives, and when the time comes when our steps may falter, our minds wander, may our spirits be free to soar.

The word "elder" still has a real meaning in many societies where it's associated with experience and the concept of wisdom. Getting older, however, doesn't necessarily mean becoming wiser. Many people are wise when they're chronologically young, and there are certainly many middle aged and older people who carry not a hint of wisdom (but perhaps have never really been encouraged to manifest it). But the opportunities for growing into that stage of development where consciousness and awareness is our natural way of being, where we've become less and less susceptible to rushing torrents of emotions and raging hormones, are here now. The concept of being in the present moment expressed in Ram Dass' book "Be Here Now" can really be applied to this stage where living in the present moment may be just a little easier than it used to be, where it's more than a concept that resonates, but a living actuality. Be present, pay attention, live your life with integrity and you'll become an "elder" whether you intended to or not!

Interviews

any of us have heroes or heroines. It's the stuff of mythology, of novels, of poems and biographies. We recognize them in art and in music. We acknowledge them with tributes such as the Nobel prize, bestow titles upon them, erect statues to their memories. Their songs have been sung by troubadours, their sagas recited around campfires. Through various means, we celebrate them because they inspire us on some level due to their achievements or because of the nobility of their character.

Some have directly touched our lives while others we know of only through their stories. Often we've internalized those stories and they become teachers for us, just as much as those with whom we've had direct contact. At times they can influence the direction of our lives. The people who have appeared on these pages are representative of people in every community. They have taken their place as elders because they have taken on the way of living responsibly, with consciousness, compassion and creativity.

We are all mirrors for each other. Sometimes we are presented with ones that reflect our less admirable aspects in order for us to recognize similar qualities within ourselves, enabling us to see those parts of ourselves more clearly. But we can also recognize those mirrors that are held up for us to see that say, "look at that wonderful human being" and realize that is what the future could hold for us as well. It can be an important time of creativity, compassion and openness to receive and embrace what life has to offer. As you will see, life has been just as difficult and wonderful, challenging and rewarding for each of these people who have appeared in this book as it has been for all of us, but how they live their lives is like a light that illuminates.

Getting older is not necessarily a guarantee of becoming wiser or more gracious. But when we encounter those around us who are not only older but really represent the kind of people we respect and admire, who inspire us by who they are, we are the recipients of a gift. I have shared some of my gifts with you in these pages through people who live their lives consciously. I'd like to share, as well, my strong feeling that now is the time to take our own place as thoughtful, compassionate beings who have had a lifetime of experiences and who are ready to realize themselves more fully by living a more mindful life through a state of heightened awareness.

Dale Amburn
Born in Farmland, Indiana - 1928

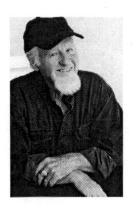

hen I first started thinking about the people I found inspiring because of the way they utilized their life experiences, Dale was one of the first people who came to mind. I met him close to thirty years ago when he first arrived in Taos and was in the midst of a major life change. After many years of operating his own design studio of graphic, architectural, interior and package design and illustration, as well as painting and teaching professional art at Indiana/Purdue Universities' regional campus of Fort Wayne, Indiana, he was diagnosed with multiple sclerosis in his early forties. At that time he made the conscious commitment to take control of his own health and proceeded to become involved in the healing effects of proper and healthy diet. He spent a great deal of time and energy researching food and the importance of proper intake of vitamins and minerals, eliminating foods he knew to be detrimental to his health, using whatever means and information he found applicable to keep the disease from which he suffered under control. The more he became involved in nutrition, the more he had to share with others and began the work that continues to be an important part of his life today.

Seven years later, having exhausted his financial resources, but regaining his health, he found himself achieving recognition once again when the city of Santa Fe, New Mexico, a place renowned for its population of artists, selected one of his paintings for its annual poster. Just past fifty and successfully controlling what could have been a crippling disease, he again began his career, in a new place, which was to include nutritional counseling as well as his art.

Still painting full time, he spends much of his time and energy helping to heal others. He strongly believes thoughts need to be integrated and be kept in touch with the body. His own way of being in the world is an example of that unification, paying attention to all aspects and actively concerned with that integration in his daily life.

He's now working with various people, providing guidance and counseling, and continues his art projects. His latest is a series of paintings that he calls, "book of wisdom, the book of knowledge, the book of philosophy – and the fourth one (symbolized by the naked man who throws the book down, knowing that everything comes from there …) the universal well of knowledge."

Dale is handsome and fit and now, in his mid-seventies, has the same energy level he's maintained since I first met him. He's articulate and direct, having very little patience (he says) with anything less than what is authentic. Part of his philosophy is that thoughts, as well as material things, can provide a good deal of "garbage." This is reflected in his beautiful home, which is kept deliberately simple, with no adornments except his paintings on the wall. Keeping his mind and personal surroundings clear of clutter is an obvious part of his life.

He continues his long time commitment to health, saying, "I'm healthier, in better shape, have more energy and am more focused then ever before."

Helen Abramowitz
Born in New York City, NY - 1912

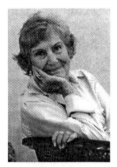

*Z*thought it was a fun thing to have become an artist's model at sixty-five, but I was the younger of the two models for a painter who was in Taos during the summer of 2000 on a Wurlitzer Foundation grant. The other model was Helen who was in her late eighties. For several years I had seen Helen working out at the spa and we always smiled, said hello, and had a few small exchanges. But it wasn't until we went out for lunch with Marjory Reid, the painter who was using us as subjects in her summer painting project, that we made a connection that put me in touch with the person whom I have found to be so inspirational, not only to me, but to the many friends whose lives she has touched.

Her spirit is incredibly uplifting, and although she has recently suffered a major loss through the death of her grandson, she still radiates the positive energy that is her hallmark. She is warm, outgoing and gracious, a reflection of an attitude that has carried her through the almost ninety years of life's pleasures and pains.

A native New Yorker and professional businesswoman, Helen's move to the small town of Taos, New Mexico was quite different from that of just a visit another person from her milieu might have made. It came about because her daughter had settled there and was raising a family. For Helen, it was a major life style change, made possible by an earlier visit with her daughter who was then living in San Lucas, a small island off Lake Atitlan in Guatemala in the 1970's. It was an experience that had great impact upon her life. Living in a small hut on the side of a mountain, using outdoor bathroom facilities, shopping in the market reached by a daily trek into town, preparing food over an open cook fire became her everyday life. Her contact with the local indigenous people and intimacy with a specific family put her in touch with another way of life with a different perspective. Then came a major earthquake and she saw firsthand how people had to cope with destruction and turmoil. Her appreciation of the culture and the environment was enhanced through her innate feelings of care and compassion, which were further honed during this stay.

She feels that this experience made her better equipped to make the shift in lifestyle, which included making wood fires and hauling water, in her new life in Taos when she was in her sixties. She also claims that because she remembers gaslights and horse and buggies, she understands the concept of change, so it wasn't hard to make the transition from a sophisticated life in New York to a more basic life in the mountains of northern New Mexico.

Now living in a home where cooking and entertaining her friends and family is part of her everyday life, she has made room for other activities as well. She still volunteers at the local hospital and museum and works out daily at the spa. The trees she planted from seed when she first moved into the house are large now, yielding a beautiful crop of apricots every year.

Helen's smile is a twinkling one and plays across her face like the ripples on the surface of a lake. If this is the face she presents to the outside world, it is a beautiful one, but only because of the place from which it comes. Her strength and determination to live a full life, to keep herself fit mentally, spiritually and physically are testimony to the values she had since childhood when afflicted with polio. She thinks it's a challenge not to be afraid of things, but to learn from them and states firmly "I refuse to give up" and says "I love change – it makes life interesting."

Pat Stallcup
Born in Frost, Texas - 1920

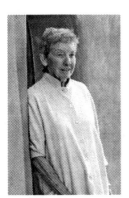

t the time I met Pat she and her husband, Bill, were both attending aerobics classes faithfully, working out three times a week as part of a core group of devotees of a class which used to be known as "Forever Fit." The people in the class range from those in their fifties to those in their eighties, all of whom work at their own pace. Although Pat no longer attends classes, she still works out on her own and keeps active at home, gardening, keeping her beautiful Southwestern style adobe house and creating sculpture and paintings on wood. Her work, done in the primitive style of northern New Mexico, reflects her artistic interest and creativity, which she produces for the pleasure she receives in the doing.

Coming from a poor and broken family in rural Texas, she didn't see much opportunity for continuing education until an adjunct professor at SMU heard about Pat and was convinced she had all the qualifications for college and helped her attain a scholarship. After graduation at twenty from SMU, where she majored in biology and received her master's degree, she did lab work for the game and fish department at a time when few women were involved in that field.

Married to a fellow graduate in 1942, Pat soon found herself spending that part of her life being the wife of an administrator at a major university, raising her five children and putting her own career on the back burner. When she felt comfortable that the responsibility of raising young children was pretty much over, she began to explore other things that were meaningful to her.

On a visit to Spain, she visited the Prado museum, which features the work of Goya as well as other renowned Spanish artists. She says of that visit that it "blew my mind," and sparked her interest in both art and the study of the Spanish language. Being in her late sixties was irrelevant to beginning a new field of study, not with a career in mind, but in following her heart, stimulating her mind and her spirit. This new focus on art and languages was an entrée to another part of self-exploration, something that continues as part of her present stage of life.

Her focus has always been inward, rather than outward. She offers a quotation from Nadine Gordimer, an African writer, from "None to Accompany Me" – "An exaltation, solitude, would come over her. Everyone ends up moving alone toward the self."

Bill Stallcup
Born in Dallas, Texas – 1920

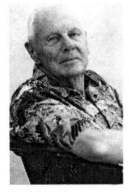

*B*ill and Pat moved to Taos full time in 1989, when Bill became director of the SMU program at nearby Fort Burgwin where he worked for the next three years after his retirement from the main university campus in Dallas. Ensconced in their new (old) adobe home in Llano Quemado, just south of Taos, they set about making a home for themselves, fixing up their house, planting beautiful lawns and flower gardens, always doing their own work, both inside and out (a metaphor for the way they live their lives).

"We've always been physically active, I believe," he says, and when Pat found the spa in 1992 they both joined, although he admits that in the beginning he was "kind of lukewarm." However he still participates in the three times a week aerobic exercise program that he began a couple of years after they joined. Earlier on, he had developed high blood pressure and finds that the cardio vascular activity is of major importance in maintaining his health and well-being. He is committed to keeping himself active and fit on all levels and his energy is outstanding, probably greater than most people a good deal younger than he. When he was teaching at SMU he ran, but found out he could do other things to keep physically fit. That's when he became more open to an exercise program.

Bill grew up in Dallas, Texas during a time of poor economy, and like Pat, was sponsored for a full scholarship at SMU where he, too, graduated at twenty with a degree in biology. After graduate school, Bill spent the next forty years teaching, first Biological Sciences and then in administration as Associate Dean in Humanities and Sciences. As an administrator, he became Associate Provost, then Vice President and Provost, and then President of SMU for a year. But all during those administrative years he always considered himself primarily a teacher.

His lifetime of dedication to service and the search for honesty in his daily life is reflected in his personal integrity which is so easily recognizable, for it is fed not by ego satisfaction but from a highly developed sense of values. Since his college years, he has been interested in service. He feels that "humans are the only animals who can choose to serve," and recalls giving a speech for a high school graduating class which had inscribed over the door to the building "Enter to learn, go forth to serve." It's the way he feels about his life.

Ted Egri
Born in New York City, N.Y. - 1913

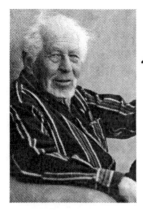

*I*n the spring of 1997, when I was in the mode of rediscovering my self, one of the first things that I became aware of was the strong desire to sculpt once again, something I had laid aside for almost thirty years. It led me, without much thought, to seek out a well-known sculptor in the town where I lived, whose work was as monumental as he was well known. I knew him to be not only an artist, but a kind, intelligent man, interested in the community in which had had lived since his arrival in the 1950's. However, it wasn't until I drove over to his house and studio with its spectacular view of the sacred Taos Mountain, and asked if he would consider taking me on as his student, that we made the connection that would establish our deep and continuing friendship.

In the many hours of grinding my pieces I found meditation, in the conversations we held together I found philosophical discussions, in seeing him down on his knees with a welding torch I found admiration, and in his never ending need to express himself in new ways, I found inspiration. Approaching his mid-eighties, he was vital, aware, interested in everything around him, still fascinated by people and their character, their foibles, their problems, their charm, their warmth, all reflections of his own character. Although he had a lifetime of experiences behind him, he was open to new ones, just as he was forever searching for new forms of creative expression.

With a background in art since childhood, he feels that his real recognition as an artist came years later through sculpture. While teaching painting at the Kansas City Art Institute, he felt great frustration at his limited ability to depict his feelings about the gross injustice of the hanging of the black men who were known as the "Martinsville Seven," followed by similar feelings of outrage when another group of black men known as the "Trenton Six" were arrested for a crime they were unjustly accused of. He found that his sculpting not only provided the physical involvement that intuitively he knew he needed to express his anger, but was a form that was to evolve as his vehicle for artistic expression that was to go beyond moral and political boundaries.

In 1950 the Egri's moved to Taos, New Mexico in the mountains of northern New Mexico while it was still a small community with no traffic lights, few paved roads and not many art galleries. Most people knew each other and the sense of familiarity was a prevalent part of that life. Ted and his wife, Kit, soon became well known in the community. The move brought with it a development of statements through sculpture, reflecting his fascination with all that he encounters and his constant search for new ways to express his ever-expanding horizons from the smallest insect to the conceptual understanding of the universe.

Not only does he carry an awareness that finds expression through his art and through the ongoing processing of new ideas that spring eternally from his ever-active mind, but is always mindful of his body as well, taking care of it and paying attention to what he needs to do for himself. His morning walks not only provide the exercise he feels he requires, but is a time of focus. It's a time when he can start the day with new eyes and finds new sources of inspiration. Ted is of the firm opinion that "stress poisons the system" and thinks instead of new creative ideas, rather than let worry and stress take over.

Ann St. John Hawley
Born in Ancon, Panama Canal Zone - 1919

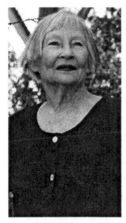

The photograph that Ann has on the mantle of her adobe fireplace is of Eleanor King, a modern dancer who lived in New Mexico for many years. It was taken when the dancer was in her late eighties or early nineties. In a traditional dancer's pose, she displays the exceptional style and grace belying her years with that special sense of timelessness that transcends the turning of pages on a calendar. This photo has a great deal of meaning to Ann, and obviously is a great inspiration to her. Now approaching her mid-eighties herself, Ann began dance lessons when she was five years old, and still dances as a continuing part of her life.

When her father, a surgeon in the army, was stationed in the Philippines, she was home schooled and was exposed to poetry and art through her mother who always encouraged her. But it was later when she was back in Washington where her father was teaching at Walter Reed Medical School that she "fell in love with dance" when she was in junior high school and knew that's what she wanted to do for the rest of her life. Her mother always emphasized finding "spirit in dance" rather than just form and this recognition of finding "spirit" in art, as well as in her daily life, is reflected in all that she does. Graduated from Northwestern University in Evanston, Ill. with a degree in theater, she became married while her husband was still in medical school. Although she raised six children, in Ann's view she was "always an artist." While she was actively involved in her family, she took classes in singing, clay, silkscreen and other art courses and, as always, dance.

Much of Ann's expression has been in the form of painting, her preferred form of art in which she incorporates her love of dance. This is why Butoh, a form of Japanese dance which she feels expresses a feeling of freedom, has played such a major role in her painting. Her lively mind is always exploring new art forms, including drumming and now the recorder. Recently she built a large studio on her property situated high on a hill with its stunning view of the Taos Mountains, just a short walk from her house, a gift she gave to herself.

Artist, dancer, mother and grandmother, Ann still finds time to attend the art openings and poetry readings of her friends. But her life is dedicated to her art and she is experienced enough to use her time wisely and conserve her energy for what's important to her. There are frequent exhibits of her work at various galleries in Taos and Santa Fe. Freedom of expression is a constant in her life, something she is has been forever seeking and manifesting through her work and her being in the world.

Her spirit is reflected in all she does, from her delightful sense of humor to her heightened state of awareness and sense of self. She continues to do the work she loves and says, "You have to have a certain amount of energy and good feeling in order to live joyfully and to live with abandon and good feeling." If this is her philosophy, it not only comes from her heart and her mind – she personifies it in all that she does. It's who she is.

To laugh often and much;

to win the respect of intelligent people and

the affection of children;

to earn the appreciation of honest critics

and endure the betrayal of false friends;

to appreciate beauty;

to find the best in others;

to leave the world a bit better, whether by

a healthy child, a garden patch or a

redeemed social condition;

to know even one life has breathed easier

because you have lived.

This is to have succeeded.

RALPH WALDO EMERSON (1803-1882)

Glossary

AWARE – Middle English IWAR Old English GEWAR
  Archaic – Watchful, wary
AWARENESS – Having or showing realization, perception or
knowledge Synonym – Cognizant – Knowledge of some
  thing. Aware – vigilance in observing or alertness in
  drawing inferences
COMPASSION – French – COMPATI – to sympathize, to
  bear, suffer, sympathetic
  consciousness of others' distress with a desire to alleviate it
CONSCIOUSNESS – Quality or state of being aware
  a. Especially of something within oneself
  b. State of being conscious of an external object, state or fact
  Mind – The totality of conscious state of individual
  The upper level of mental life of which the person is aware
  as contrasted with un-conscious processes
FIT – Suitable by nature or by art
  Adapted to environment so as to be capable of surviving
  And also transmit genotype to reproductive offspring
FITNESS – (Noun – since 1580) – Quality or state of being fit
HOLISTIC (Adjective – since 1926) – Relating to or concerned
  with Wholes or complete systems, rather than dissection
  into parts
  Concerned with complete systems
  Holistic medicine attempts to treat both mind and body
  Ecology views man and environment as a single system more
  than the sum of the parts
HOLY – Akin to Old English HAL – (Whole)
  Worthy of complete devotion as one perfect in goodness and
  righteousness or devoted entirely to the Deity

INSPIRE – (Verb) Middle French – Spirare – To breathe
   To influence, move or guide by divine or supernatural
   inspiration
   To exert an animating, exalting, enlivening influence on,
   Impel, motivate, affect
INSPIRATION – (noun, 14th century)
   A divine influence or action on a person believed to
   qualify him or her to receive and communicate sacred
   revelation
   The action or power of moving the intellect or emotions
   (also – the act of drawing in – the drawing of air into
   the lungs)
   An inspiring agent or influence
PERSPECTIVE – French – prospetto – view, prospect
   Middle Latin – Perspectivus – of sight – optical
   To look through – see clearly
   (French – per-through- and specere – to look)
   Technique of representing on a plane or curved surface
   The spatial relation of objects as they might appear to
   The eye
   Representation in and drawing of parallel lines as they
   Would appear to the eye
POINT OF VIEW – Interrelation in which subject or its parts are
   mentally viewed
   A visible scene
   A mental view or prospect
   Capacity to view things in their true relations or
   Relative importance
REVEAL – Middle English – Revelen – Uncover
   To make known through divine inspiration
   To make something (secret or hidden) publically or
   generally known
   To open up to view or display
SHIFT – Old English – Sciftan – To divide/arrange
   To exchange for or replace by another
   To change place, position, or direction – move
   To change direction
   To assume responsibility (has to shift for themselves)
   To go through a change
   To become changed

A change in emphasis, attitude
A removal from one person or thing to another – to
transfer
TRANSFORM – (verb) – Middle English
Latin – Transformare (to form)
A change in composition or structure
A change in outward form or appearance
A change in character or condition
Or to become transformed
TRANSFORMATIONAL (Adjective – 1894) – of, relating to, or
Characterized by or concerned with transformation
(especially linguistic transformation)
WELL-BEING – (noun 1613) – the state of being happy, healthy
or prosperous - welfare
WHOLE – Middle English - HOOL (healthy, unhurt, entire)
Old English – HAL – Akin to old German HEIL – healthy,
Unhurt
Free of defect or Impairment – Intact
Physically sound and healthy
Mentally and emotionally sound
Having all its proper parts and components
Constituting the total sum of undiminished entirety
Synonyms – entire, total, all

Index

Order Form

You may purchase additional copies of this book from your local book-store or from:

Toll-free credit card phone orders: 800-929-7889 (Visa & MC)
Toll-free Fax orders: 877-520-4890
Postal Orders: Paloma Blanca Press, PO Box 1751, Taos NM 87571
Order Online: www.FiftyandBeyond.com
Please copy this form for fax and mail orders.

Please send _____ **copies of** *Fifty and Beyond: New Beginnings in Health and Well-Being* **to:**

Name: _____

Address: _____

City: _____ **State/Province:** _____

Zip/Postal Code: _____ **Country:** _____

Telephone: _____

Email address: _____

Sales tax: Please add 7% for books shipped to New Mexico addresses.

Shipping by air:
US: $3.95 for first book and $2.00 for each additional book
International: $8.75 US for first book; $4.75 US for each additional book

Signed copy (no extra charge) Autograph to read (please print legibly!):

_____

☐ Payment: ☐ Check (payable to Paloma Blanca Press) ☐ Credit card:
☐ Visa ☐ MasterCard ☐ AMEX ☐ Discover
Card number:_____
Name on card: _____ Exp. Date: _____
Signature: _____

Look for Susanna Starr's next book: *Fifty and Beyond: New Life Beginnings*
ATTENTION: ORGANIZATIONS, EDUCATIONAL INSTITUTIONS, AND INDUSTRY PUBLICATIONS: Quantity discounts are available on bulk purchases of this book for reselling, educational purposes, subscription incentives, gifts, or fund raising. Special books or book excerpts can also be created to fit specific needs. For information, please contact Paloma Blanca Press, Special Sales Dept., POB 1751, Taos NM 87571 877-520-4890.

LaVergne, TN USA
18 September 2009
158317LV00001B/57/A